For Butterworth Heinemann:

Commissioning Editor: Mary Seager
Development Editor: Catharine Steers
Project Controller: Morven Dean
Designer: Andy Chapman
Illustration Manager: Bruce Hogarth

The Really Useful Handbook of

Reptile Husbandry

Caroline Gosden VN

Veterinary Nurse, Animal Care/VN Lecturer, UK

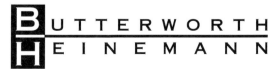

BUTTERWORTH HEINEMANN

An Imprint of Elsevier Science Limited

Edinburgh • London • New York • Oxford • Philadelphia • St Louis • Sydney • Toronto • 2004

BUTTERWORTH-HEINEMANN
An imprint of Elsevier Science Limited

First published 2004

ISBN 0 7506 5443 0

British Library Cataloguing in Publication Data
A catalogue record for this book is available from the British Library

Library of Congress Cataloging in Publication Data
A catalog record for this book is available from the Library of
Congress

Veterinary knowledge is constantly changing. Standard safety
precautions must be followed, but as new research and clinical
experience broaden our knowledge, changes in treatment and drug
therapy may become necessary or appropriate. Readers are advised
to check the most current product information provided by the
manufacturer of each drug to be administered to verify the
recommended dose, the method and duration of administration, and
contraindications. It is the responsibility of the practitioner, relying on
experience and knowledge of the patient, to determine dosages and
the best treatment for each individual patient. Neither the Publisher nor
the author assumes any liability for any injury and/or damage to
persons or property arising from this publication.
The Publisher

 your source for books,
journals and multimedia
in the health sciences

www.elsevierhealth.com

Printed in China

The
publisher's
policy is to use
**paper manufactured
from sustainable forests**

CONTENTS

The CD-ROM accompanying this text includes blank history forms, a quiz based on the information in the book, an iguana food chart and searchable illustrations of reptiles.

PREFACE

This book is designed to be of use to any establishment or individual who, from time to time, may need instant information on how to care for commonly kept reptiles or amphibians.

The idea first occurred to me when I was teaching exotic animal husbandry to veterinary nursing students. It quickly became apparent that the majority of veterinary practices treat reptiles only on the odd occasion. Because of this, knowledge of their husbandry and illnesses is limited and there is not the incentive to spend a lot of time researching information that may only be used once or twice a year.

The most common reason for illness amongst reptiles is inappropriate husbandry. I have found that detailed questioning about the housing and feeding will usually reveal the cause of the problem.

This is a book that is quick and easy to use and that will assist in establishing the cause of an illness (although not in its treatment as there are already enough books that cover this aspect), or better still, how to prevent problems occurring in the first place.

1 BLANK HISTORY FORMS AND EXPLANATION OF THE QUESTIONS

These forms can be copied and given to owners to fill in, or used as a prompt to question the owner and get the information verbally. Either way they will reveal detailed information about the way the animal is being kept and hopefully pinpoint any errors.

Behind each form is an explanation as to why each question is being asked and tips/advice as to what is or is not appropriate.

You will get the hang of it once you start reading! It is worth pointing out that some answers may require further questioning. (See the comments in the self test section.)

HISTORY

SNAKES & LIZARDS

ANIMAL'S DETAILS

Name _____

Species (and subspecies if known) _____

Sex _____

Where did you get it from? _____

Approximate age _____

How long have you had it? _____

When and with what was it last wormed? _____

HOUSING

VIVARIUM

What is the vivarium made of? _____

What are its measurements? _____

How is ventilation provided? _____

LIGHTING

Is there any UV provision? (State type of tube used and

how frequently it is changed) _____

How high above the substrate is the UV positioned? _____

_____

Is there a spotlight/basking light? (State type and wattage) _____

_____

Does the spotlight have a guard around it? _____

For how long are the lights on each day?

Summer _____

Winter _____

HEATING

What type of heater is used? _____

Does it have a guard around it? _____

Is it connected to a thermostat? _____

State the background temperatures: Summer   Winter

Day _____

Night _____

Do you use min./max. thermometers? _____

What is the temperature under the spotlight/basking light? _____

Is all the heating and lighting equipment at the same end of the vivarium? _____

What is the temperature difference between the hot end and the cool end? _____

HUMIDITY

What is the humidity? _____

Is there a humidity gauge? _____

How is it provided? _____

DÉCOR

What substrate is used? _____

How deep is the substrate? _____

How frequently is the vivarium cleaned out? _____

What cleaning solution is used? _____

Describe the hide box/es _____

Is there a covered, damp, moss/peat container? _____

What other items of décor are there? (Rocks, branches, drain pipes, plastic or real plants, etc.) _____

FEEDING

List **all** food items including quantity and frequency *or* complete a diet sheet. **See Appendix I** (If fruit & vegetables list each type)

_____

_____

_____

_____

_____

_____

_____

_____

_____

_____

How often is the animal fed? _____

What supplements are provided and how often? _____

_____

If feeding with insects, how do you ensure the supplement is delivered? _____

What are the insects fed on? _____

What size is the water container? _____

SOCIAL GROUPING

What other individuals of the same or different species share the accommodation? _____

How many are there of each and of what sex? _____

Do they tend to mix with or ignore each other? _____

_____

Is there at least one hide per individual? _____

COOLING DOWN

Please describe fully the process of cooling down, length of cooling and warming back up. _____

_____

_____

_____

_____

_____

_____

_____

ANY OTHER COMMENTS

_____

_____

_____

_____

_____

_____

_____

_____

EXPLANATION OF QUESTIONS
SNAKES & LIZARDS

*[THIS SECTION ALSO INCLUDES SOME GENERAL DETAILS
RELEVANT TO THE OTHER REPTILES AND AMPHIBIANS]*

ANIMAL'S DETAILS

Where did you get it from?

Was it a pet shop, private breeder, friend, rescued, wild caught,
captive bred, etc. This can have a bearing on the problem; for
example, if it was wild caught it will probably be stressed for
several weeks or months after capture and will undoubtedly
have a parasite burden, whereas if it came from a breeder or
friend the owner may have some knowledge of its history. Ask
for details of how it was being cared for previously.

Approximate age

There are fairly obvious reasons for asking this because, for
example, if the animal is very young then congenital abnormality
should be considered; if old it may be just old age. However, the
age may well be unknown or, at best, approximate.

How long have you had it?

This will allow you to decide whether previous owner history is
relevant. Also, bear in mind that newly acquired animals may
become stressed for several weeks, purely due to being
relocated.

When and with what was it last wormed?

All species, whether captive bred or wild caught, should be
wormed regularly, that is approximately twice a year. The most

widely used wormer is Panacur 10% solution, 1 ml/kg for most species.

HOUSING

The following text gives guidelines, however, for specific species' requirements refer either to the species sheets at the back of this section or a book that deals with the subject.

VIVARIUM
What is the vivarium made of?

Glass and plastic. These are waterproof but do not retain the heat well and the animal may feel insecure if most of the sides are not covered.

Fibreglass. This is also waterproof but, again, does not retain the heat well.

Wood. This is heat retaining and provides a sense of security; however, it should have a water-resistant finish by being, for example, regularly coated with varnish or covered in melamine, and all the joins should be filled with a waterproof sealant.

> **Tip** It doesn't matter what sort of varnish or sealant is used provided it is thoroughly dry and the fumes are completely evaporated before putting the animal in.

What are its measurements?

There are no 'hard and fast' rules for this; my own view is that the vivarium should be as large as possible in order to provide adequate environmental stimulation. Obviously, the greater the number of individuals the larger it should be. It should also reflect the natural habits of the animal, e.g. tall for arboreal species, or deep to allow for a thick layer of substrate for those that burrow.

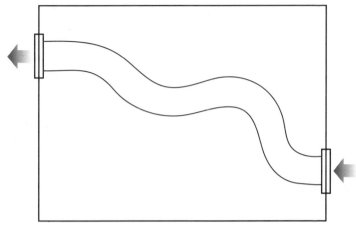

Fig. 1.1 Diagram showing through—flow of air. Adapted with permission, from the Prevetinary Nursing Textbook by Masters and Bowden, Butterworth Heinemann (2001).

How is ventilation provided?
Good ventilation is essential. To provide an adequate through-flow of air there should be ventilation panels at both the top and bottom. (See Fig. 1.1)

LIGHTING
Is there any UV provision?
Many reptiles use UV to synthesise Vitamin D (snakes are one of the main exceptions). There are two main ways of providing this:

1   Pure UV lights (often referred to as 'black lights'). These are very strong and should only be turned on for short periods of time, e.g. 15–30 minutes two or three times a day.
2   Full spectrum lights. These are more popular now and as the name implies, they provide the full spectrum of light and can be left on all day.

Black lights emit UV for their entire life span but many of the full-spectrum lights only emit UV for approximately 6 months, although they will continue to provide illumination for considerably longer.

How high above the substrate is the UV positioned?

UV readings are highest nearer to the tube and decline rapidly further away. At a distance of approximately 2 feet (60 cm) they are almost negligible. Therefore, the tube should be placed either near the substrate or in a position that allows the animal to get close to it, such as above a basking rock or near a branch, whichever is most suitable for the species in question.

Is there a spotlight/basking light?

For many species basking in the sun is a natural way of thermoregulation and they will need to express this behaviour in captivity. A slight increase in the temperature under the spotlight is sufficient for some species but for others, primarily those from desert areas, a temperature of 40°C is not unusual. The many different ways of providing this include ordinary household incandescent bulbs, infrared bulbs, ceramic bulbs, spotlights etc. The appropriateness of what is being used should be judged against the circumstances.

Does the spotlight/basking light have a guard around it?

If there is **any** possibility of the animal coming into physical contact with the bulb it **must** be covered with a wire mesh guard. Serious burns can result from unprotected lighting or heating equipment. (See Fig. 1.2)

For how long are the lights on each day?

You need to check:

- whether the day length is appropriate.
- that everything that provides illumination goes off at night.
- whether it would be more natural (given the geographical origin of the species) for spotlight/basking lights to go on and off during the day, mimicking the natural pattern of the sun.

9

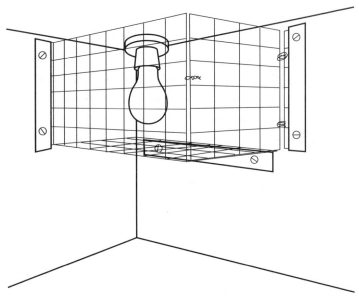

Fig. 1.2 Diagram showing wire mesh guard

(Obviously, it is not possible to precisely copy the sun's pattern but an example might be to have two or three periods of perhaps an hour when the light is off.)

In the wild many species would experience seasonal variation in the day length and this should be reflected in captivity with a gradual decline in the length of time the lighting is on for during the winter and reversing this in the spring. Reducing the temperature, that is the wattage of the spotlight/basking light, might also be appropriate. If proper hibernation conditions are needed then the total absence of light should be considered.

HEATING
What type of heater is used?
There are numerous types available, for example a tubular greenhouse heater, which is usually attached to the back wall approximately 6 inches (15 cm) above the substrate level, or a

heat plate/ceramic heater which is usually attached to the ceiling. As a general rule I do not recommend using hot rocks at all or heat mats *within* the vivarium for two reasons:

1　They require the reptile to make direct contact with them and can therefore cause burns.
2　They will only provide heat in their immediate vicinity and are not designed to heat large spaces.

Does it have a guard around it?

Most of these heaters will get extremely hot and will burn the animal if it comes into contact with it. A wire mesh guard should cover the heater, thus preventing the animal sitting on it or curling up around it.

Is it connected to a thermostat?

This is essential if the temperature within the vivarium is to be controlled.

State the background temperatures

What you are looking for here is a difference in the ambient temperature of approx. 5–8°C between the daytime and nighttime for the majority of the year (summer) and (for the reasons already mentioned above in the lighting section), you also need to know whether a cooling down period is provided (winter). The length and temperature of the cooling will depend on the species; however, as a general rule there are a few guidelines that should be followed:

1　The change from summer to winter temperatures should be gradual (approx. 2°C per week).
2　Once the nighttime temperature reaches the correct level the day time temperature should continue to fall until it is the same as the night, so that a constant temperature is maintained for the duration.

3   (Obviously) the reduction in lighting and heating should
     occur simultaneously.

N.B. It is worth mentioning here that during cooling down and
hibernation, disturbance should be kept to an absolute minimum.

Do you use min./max. thermometers?

If this is not the case it is impossible to accurately gauge the
temperature fluctuation within the vivarium, especially at night. It
is best to have one thermometer at each end of the vivarium.

What is the temperature under the spotlight/basking light?

Again, this has already been discussed previously in the section on
lighting but it is mentioned here to emphasise the importance of
being aware of the temperature that the spotlight/basking light is
creating.

Is all the heating and lighting equipment at the same end of the vivarium?

In order to create a 'hot end' and a 'cool end' it is necessary to
place all equipment that generates heat (however minimal) at the
same end of the vivarium. This is explained more fully below. One
exception to this is that in large vivariums, or those housing desert
animals, it may be necessary to have daylight tubes covering the
whole or majority of the length of the vivarium (see Fig. 1.3).

What is the temperature difference between the hot end and the cool end?

In the wild a reptile will thermo-regulate, in other words move
into a sunny or hot position when it needs to warm up, then
move off when it has achieved its preferred body temperature
(PBT). This facility should be provided in captivity. In its simplest
form this is done by making one end of the vivarium a few

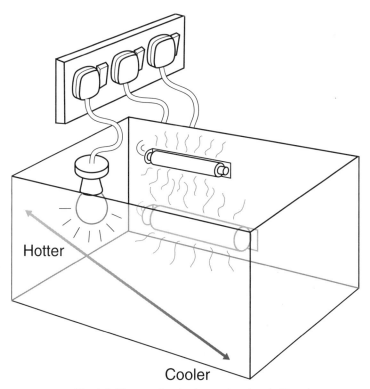

Hotter

Cooler

Fig. 1.3 Diagram showing hot and cool end of housing

degrees hotter than the other (see above); however, this should
be elaborated upon by providing a basking spot, as already
discussed in the lighting section, and also cool areas dotted
around the vivarium. These can be pots or containers with
dampened moss or peat inside them, clay pipes, rocks, or a
deep substrate layer into which the animal can burrow.

HUMIDITY
What is the humidity?
Again, this should be similar to that experienced by the animal in
its natural habitat. It is important to get this right as too high a
humidity may cause blistering on the skin, particularly with
snakes, whilst too low may cause difficulty with sloughing.

Is there a humidity gauge?

It is surprising how many people will tell me what the humidity is but when asked what type of gauge they use say they don't have one. How can the humidity be known without using a gauge?! (See Fig. 1.4)

How is it provided?

There are several ways of providing humidity, the most common being to use a spray bottle two or three times daily. It should preferably be with warm water so that the temperature within the vivarium is not affected too much. Other methods that help to contribute to the overall humidity are: dampened peat containers, real plants, or placing a water container on the heater (although this method is prone to ending up with most of the water anywhere other than in the container and is not one that I recommend). Another more sophisticated method is to have a misting device that simulates gentle rainfall.

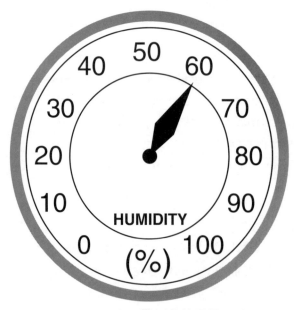

Fig. 1.4 Humidity gauge

> **Tip** This is only possible with large vivariums as smaller ones will quickly become saturated

DÉCOR

What substrate is used?

Points to consider here are whether the substrate is:

- suitable for the level of humidity, that is it will not go mouldy or soggy in a humid environment. I like to use potting compost (and being an environmentally aware sort, the type without peat) or bark chips from the garden centre. There are alternatives available from specialist reptile shops, such as orchid bark, but these are rather expensive. For fairly dry environments I do use substrate from the reptile shops, e.g. beech bark or corn chip.

> **Tip** Preferably the type without pine needles as the smell can be rather overpowering for the reptile

- suitable for an animal that likes to burrow or hide.
- likely to lead to impaction if ingested. A certain amount of substrate will inevitably be ingested during feeding and the smaller the granule size, the more likely impaction becomes. There are substrates available that the manufacturers claim to be digestible but even these can cause a problem if ingested in sufficient quantity.

How deep is the substrate?

For burrowing or ground dwelling species the substrate needs to be deep enough to allow this behaviour.

How frequently is the vivarium cleaned out?

This obviously depends on the species, the size of the vivarium and number of individuals. It is not usually necessary to perform a total clean-out frequently provided that spot cleaning is carried out daily; indeed, too frequent total cleaning may cause the animal unnecessary stress. However, there is no excuse for a vivarium to smell and if an air change (blowing fresh air through the vivarium with a small fan etc.) does not alleviate the smell then a total clean-out should be done.

What cleaning solution is used?

For most vivariums an antibacterial soap should be used at the very least and preferably a disinfectant suitable for reptile use such as Trigene or Tamodene-E (specifically for reptiles). This is particularly important if total clean-outs occur infrequently. However, if cleaning of a particular area or item happens regularly and there is no risk of contamination, ordinary soap or just hot water may suffice every so often.

Describe the hide box/es

If the vivarium contains a single animal there should be two hides, one at each end of the vivarium, in order that the animal does not have to compromise its thermoregulatory behaviour, and there should be a minimum of one hide per animal where there is more than one individual. The hide should be just large enough for the animal to fit into comfortably; too big and it will not feel secure. It does not have to be an elaborate structure; very often a cardboard box with a hole cut into it (just large enough for the animal to fit through) is more than adequate. See Fig. 1.5 for types of hide/box.

Is there a covered, damp, peat/moss container?

This has three main functions as it provides:

- a cool spot for thermoregulation.
- a damp area, which will aid sloughing.

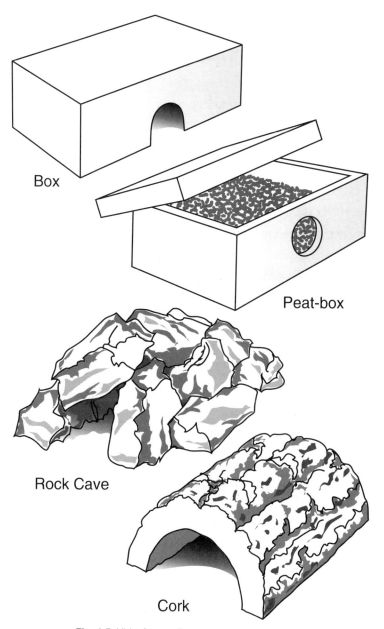

Fig. 1.5 Hides/boxes: Box, peat box, rock cave, cork

- a suitable area for females to lay eggs. This is most important as some females will retain their eggs if they feel that there is nowhere suitable for them to lay and this may result in egg binding. It is important to remember that females can produce eggs in the absence of a male although they will probably be infertile, however, the females of some species can retain viable sperm for many months or even years.

What other items of décor are there?

Some people keep reptiles, particularly snakes, in what is called the drawer system. This is a space- and time-saving way of keeping large collections and, if this system is employed, there will probably not be any other items of décor. However, I would rather see them in a more spacious enclosure with as much environmental stimulation as possible, such as that shown in Fig. 1.6

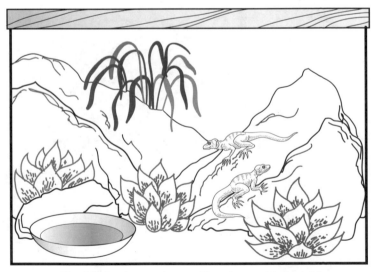

Fig. 1.6 Spacious enclosure with environmental stimulation

FEEDING

This is one of the major problem areas and the requirements of an individual species should be researched thoroughly. It is impossible to cover all aspects in sufficient depth in these pages; therefore the following will highlight only the basics and further research on individual species may be necessary.

The first two questions should be looked at in conjunction with each other to establish an overall diet. In some instances it may be more useful to substitute the blank diet sheet at Appendix 1 for these two questions.

List all food items fed and how often each is given.

- For species that are predominantly herbivorous, variety is the key. Most owners will say that they feed all kinds of fruit and vegetables but when asked to list them it is often a surprisingly short list. Many of the 'herbivores' will also eat other types of food. For example Bearded Dragons will eat seeds and insects.
- Species that are predominantly insectivorous have a limited diet in captivity but this does not usually present a problem. There are some foods that should not be given too frequently, such as waxworms because these have an extremely high fat content and may also become addictive. Like the herbivores, many of the insectivores will also enjoy other types of food. Leopard geckos, for example, may enjoy a pinkie (baby mouse) occasionally.
- Omnivorous species should also be offered a variety of food. One of the problems commonly encountered with captive omnivores is that because they are so well fed they become fussy and will often only take their favourite foods (usually the carnivorous portion of the diet). This can obviously lead to dietary problems such as too high a

protein content or obesity and every effort should be made to prevent this occurring.

- Pelleted food is available for many species, which is a useful addition to the diet but should be considered as only one constituent in a varied diet.
- As suggested above, if an animal has a particularly favourite food it should not be given too frequently as it may start to refuse to eat anything else. Some notorious examples are:
  Terrapins – prawns
  Herbivores & omnivores – bananas
  Snakes, especially Burmese pythons – chicks/chickens
- Most snakes are carnivorous and their diet, though fairly monotonous, does not usually present a problem. Refusing to feed, however, is not uncommon. Remember that a snake can survive for months, even years in some cases, without eating so, providing it is in good general body condition, there is no need to panic straight away.

There are many reasons why a snake may refuse food. **Appendix 2** shows a flow chart which details a step by step guide that may help to ascertain and rectify the problem. However, it is intended as an **initial guide** only and is by no means exhaustive, therefore expert advice may need to be considered.

How often is the animal fed?

The frequency of feeding largely depends on the amount given each time so common sense must be employed when looking at an individual's diet.

Most species do not need to be fed daily but this fact should be offset against the environmental stimulation that eating affords and therefore, for most species, daily or every other day is a good average. Snakes are the obvious exception to this and, as a general rule, the larger the snake the less frequently it should be fed, but it should be given as large a prey item as possible.

> Tip As a rough guide, the food item should be as large as the widest part of the snake's body

Some knowledge should be obtained on the do's and don'ts of feeding snakes in order to advise owners on their regime.

What supplements are provided and how often?

Any supplement should be one that is designed specifically for reptiles. There are a variety of these available: Nutrobal, Reptivite and as to how often they should be given the label will provide detailed information. Some species may benefit from additional calcium/phosphorous supplementation and again this comes in a number of forms. Needless to say over-supplementation can be equally inappropriate as insufficient.

If feeding with insects, how do you ensure the supplement is delivered?

If insects are dusted with the supplement and then released into the vivarium the supplement will quickly become dislodged, either rubbing off on the décor or substrate, or the insect will clean it off itself. Hand-feeding the reptile with some of the crickets will ensure this does not happen and also has the added advantage that the owner will know immediately if an animal is off its food.

> Tip I don't mean with the fingers here but, rather, using small plastic tweezers. (Plastic is important as the lizard will often grab the tweezers as well as the cricket.)

What are the insects fed on?

Unless they are fed a good quality diet, their nutritional content to the reptile will be negligible. There are several cricket diets available, for example 'bug grub', or a variety of fruit and vegetables can be offered. A particular favourite of mine is to give good quality fish flakes and, say, apple for moisture. One of the few exceptions to this are waxworms as these larvae when sold have already been through the gorging-themselves stage and are now ready to pupate.

> **Tip** Once bought, crickets should not be kept in the plastic tub they are sold in but transferred to a small ventilated container. Waxworms, however, can be left in their tub but should be kept in the fridge as this will delay them turning into pupae.

What size is the water container?

Some snakes will use their water bowl to help them to shed and will lie completely or partially submerged for hours. Although this behaviour is reduced when other suitable means of obtaining sufficient humidity is provided, such as a peat container, it is still preferable to allow the snake some choice.

Chelonia and many lizards do not require deep water and indeed, it may be dangerous to provide it; however, some rainforest species of lizard may need a large area in order to allow natural behaviour. (E.g. iguana, Water dragon, Tegu)

SOCIAL GROUPING

What other individuals of the same or different species share the accommodation?

Most species will tolerate company, indeed it often provides environmental stimulation (even if in the wild the species is not usually gregarious), however, it can also be detrimental and the questions you need to ask are:

Tip One notable exception are the King snakes, which will often try to eat each other if kept together.

1   Is the vivarium suitable for the number of individuals?
2   Is the mix of sexes right? Some species, such as corn snakes, will tolerate more than one male in a group whereas others, for example Leopard geckos, will not.

As a general rule I do not advocate mixing different species as it is usually difficult to get the conditions to meet the specific environmental requirements of both, a typical example of this would be water dragons & iguanas.

How many are there of each and of what sex?

[*See above.*] Sexing guidelines are as follows:

1   Snakes. For most species it is difficult to tell male from female other than by probing. This procedure involves inserting a metal probe into the cloaca but, as the potential to injure the snake is quite high, this should only be performed by someone who is experienced in the procedure.
2   Lizards. Several factors may be taken into consideration but in most species these will not become apparent until sexual maturity is attained.
    — In some species the male may be a different colour to the female. For example the male dab-tailed lizard *maliensis* is black, the female brown.
    — The male may be larger and more stocky than the female or have more or larger body adornments: the male Jackson's chameleon has three horns but the female is hornless; the spiny crest and dewlap of the male green iguana are often larger than those of the females.
    — For many species the most reliable way is to look at the femoral pores (Fig. 1.7) which are more pronounced in the

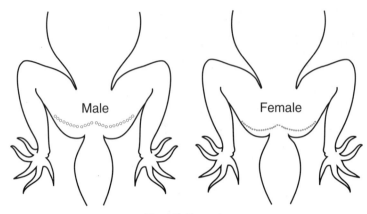

Fig. 1.7 Femoral pores

male, especially during the breeding season, e.g. Leopard gecko, Bearded Dragon.

— Some species, however, are very difficult to sex unless you are experienced, e.g. blue-tongued skink.

3   Chelonia. In the majority of tortoise species there are three characteristics to look for:

— Males often have a longer tail than females.

— The plastron (ventral shell) is often more concave in the male.

— The shape of the rear plastral lobe (see Fig. 1.8).

In some aquatic species the male has much longer claws on the forelimbs, e.g. red-eared terrapin.

Do they tend to mix with or ignore each other?
Observations as to how the individuals interact with each other is very important. If they are aggressive to each other then obviously they should be separated, but there are other less obvious signs that might indicate that the stress of being mixed is too great, such as:

• each staying at different ends of the vivarium
• giving each other a wide berth when passing

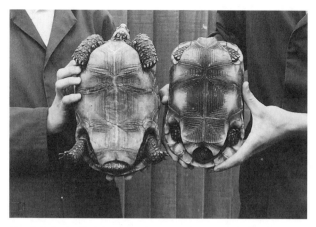

Fig. 1.8 Sexing tortoises showing rear plastral lobes. The male is on the left with the wider lobes. Adapted with permission, from the Pre-Veterinary Nursing Textbook by Masters and Bowden, Butterworth Heinemann (2001)

- one eating only when the other has finished or not eating at all
- mock attacks
- little activity during the part of the day when they should be awake

It must be stressed that there may be other reasons for these behaviours, including illness, or it may be normal behaviour for that individual.

Is there as least one hide per individual?
Even successfully mixed individuals that share a hide regularly may prefer solitude at times.

COOLING DOWN
Please explain fully the process of cooling down, length of cooling and warming up.
The first point to establish is whether the species experiences a cooling down in the wild because if it does not then it should not be subjected to it in captivity. If it does, the things to look for are:

- a gradual reduction in temperature over a few weeks until both day and night-time temperatures are the same. (The eventual temperature will vary according to species.)
- a reduction in the lighting at the same time as the temperature is being reduced. This may be achieved by reducing the wattage of the light bulbs and/or, if there are several light sources, turning one off each week.
- an appropriate length of time for the cooling down/hibernation. (Again this will vary with the species.)
- minimal disturbance during cooling down, but obviously occasional checks should be made.
- a gradual reversal of both temperature and lighting at the end of cooling, back up to the original.

Tip some species may not require a proper cooling down, rather a slight reduction in the temperature and lighting intensity, e.g. Dab-tailed lizard

Any other comments. This allows for anything that has not already been covered. It may be that the owner feels there is something else relevant, or you may like to guide them with suggestions of your own.

HISTORY

TORTOISES

[IF THE TORTOISE IS KEPT IN A VIVARIUM INSIDE THE HOUSE USE THE HISTORY FORM FOR SNAKES & LIZARDS]

ANIMAL'S DETAILS

Name _____

Species _____

Sex _____

Where did you get it from? _____

Approximate age _____

How long have you had it? _____

When and with what was it last wormed? _____

HOUSING

HOUSE

Describe the house and run. Include approximate size, construction materials and a diagram if applicable. (If there is more than one accommodation type provided, fill in a separate form for each.)

_____

_____

_____

_____

_____

_____

_____

During inclement weather is the tortoise shut in its house or does it still have access to the outside?_____

_____

LIGHTING

Is there any UV provision? (State type used and how frequently it is changed) _____

How high above 'tortoise level' is it placed? _____

Is there a spotlight/basking light? (State type & wattage) _____

For how long are the lights on each day? _____

HEATING

What type of heater is used? _____

Does it have a guard around it? _____

Is it connected to a thermostat? _____

What is the background temperature? Day _____ Night _____

What is the temperature variation between the hot and cold sections? _____

_____

What is the temperature under the spotlight/basking light? _____

What type of thermometer is used? _____

DÉCOR

What substrate is used? _____

How frequently is it cleaned out? _____

What cleaning solution is used? _____

Describe the hide box/es _____

If there is a special area for egg laying, describe it _____

_____

FEEDING

List **all** types of food items given including quantity and
frequency *or* complete a diet sheet. **See Appendix I**_____

_____

_____

_____

_____

_____

_____

State approximately how much is given on a daily basis _____
What supplements are given and how often? _____

SOCIAL GROUPING

What other individuals of the same or different species share the
accommodation? (State how many there are of each and of
what sex) _____

_____

Describe how they interact with each other_____

_____

_____

_____

HIBERNATION

If you provide a gradual cooling down prior to hibernation,
please describe the process_____

_____

_____

_____

_____

_____

For how long is food withheld prior to entering hibernation?_____
Do you worm the tortoise prior to hibernation?_____

How do you ensure adequate bodyweight prior to
hibernation?_____

_____

Describe the hibernation accommodation and siting in detail ___

_____

_____

_____

_____

_____

_____

_____

How often do you check the tortoise during hibernation? _____
At the end of hibernation do you wake the tortoise yourself or
allow it to wake up on its own? _____
If it wakes up by itself, how do you know when it has
done so? _____

_____

_____

Please describe what you do immediately the tortoise has
woken up and for the following few days _____

_____

_____

_____

_____

_____

_____

ANY OTHER COMMENTS

_____

_____

_____

_____

_____

_____

EXPLANATION OF QUESTIONS

TORTOISES

[WHERE A SPECIFIC QUESTION IS NOT EXPLAINED REFER TO THE SNAKES & LIZARDS SECTION]

HOUSING

HOUSE

Describe the house.

This should be large enough to allow the tortoise to wander about a bit when it is shut in. Height is not particularly important other than to ensure sufficient clearance above the shell and to allow freedom of movement and the provision of lighting. Adequate size will depend on the:

- size of tortoise
- number of tortoises being housed together
- length of time the tortoise is confined to the house

As far as construction goes you are looking for solid construction that is:

- strong enough to deter other animals, e.g. rats, mice, foxes
- able to withstand the weather
- able to maintain a good thermal insulation

and run.

This may vary between the whole garden or a purpose built 'rabbit run' type. The run needs to:

- be large enough to provide the tortoise with sufficient space for stimulation, such as investigating potential food sources or hiding places; escaping unwanted attention from other tortoises.

- be of solid construction, but this time to keep the tortoise in. They will dig and climb.
- prevent access to poisonous plants.

During inclement weather is the tortoise shut in its house or does it still have access to the outside?

Inclement weather for a tortoise includes anything that results in the temperature falling below about 25°C. In this country this occurs quite often, even in the summer.

If the tortoise still has access to the outside, the owner should be quite sure that it will return to its house when it gets cold. Tortoises can be irritatingly stupid about this and remain outside whilst getting progressively colder and more lethargic.

On the other hand if the tortoise is shut away it will mean that a considerable amount of time will be spent in its house and the size of the house should reflect this.

DÉCOR
Describe the area for egg laying.

Tortoises need an area for laying eggs for the same reasons as snakes and lizards. Those individuals with access to the garden may well use a flower border but they may equally well decide it is not suitable and, for those individuals that spend a considerable amount of time inside their houses, the garden may not be an option. In other words, it is advisable to provide a large, deep receptacle filled with soil or peat, whatever the circumstances.

FEEDING

List all types of food items and state approximately how often each is given.

Most (but not all) tortoises are pure herbivores, so a diet with as great a variety as possible is important. This should include a wide selection of:

- vegetables and fruit
- non-poisonous garden plants, e.g. dandelion flowers & leaves, clover flowers & leaves, groundsel, etc.
- herbs
- pelleted food, e.g. T Rex tortoise food, herbivore mix, etc.
- hay, alfalfa, grass. (For some species, e.g. the African spurred tortoise, this forms the bulk of their diet, and is, of course, more natural.)

Tip Don't forget that some foods can become addictive e.g. banana

SOCIAL GROUPING

[For sexing of tortoises, see p. 24.]

Describe how they interact with each other.
Very often the only interaction is that of mating. Males can be extraordinarily persistent about this (and not only with females) to the point where it becomes a problem and they may need to be separated in order to relieve the recipient/s of their constant (and usually unwanted) attention.

HIBERNATION

Before discussing hibernation technique it must be established if the tortoise is suitable to hibernate.
The following rules should be followed.

1 Only hibernate a species if it does so in the wild. Although other species of tortoise are becoming popular, the most commonly kept are the Mediterranean tortoises (Hermans and Spur-thighed) and these species do undergo hibernation.
2 Sick or underweight individuals should not be hibernated.

3   The smaller (younger) the tortoise is, the shorter the period
    of hibernation should be. (Many people prefer not to
    hibernate very young individuals, that is, those under about
    3 years old, but this does depend on size.)

**If you provide a gradual cooling down prior to hibernation,
please describe the process.**

You need a 'yes' in response to the first part of this question. In
the wild tortoises would use the shortening day length and
cooling temperatures as their cue to prepare for hibernation.
They need the same sort of stimulus in captivity.

Individuals that have access to the outside on a daily basis
may use the natural change in the seasons, although the
conditions in their housing must also reflect these changes.

If the tortoise is kept inside its housing, for the most part, then
the changes must be artificial. To a certain extent the timing can be
controlled by the owners so, for example, if they were going on
holiday in October and wanted the tortoise to be snug in its
hibernation by then, they could induce this state earlier than usual.

For how long is food withheld prior to hibernation?

This should be for 4–6 weeks, the time it takes for the digestive
tract to empty completely. If food is left in the system it will
ferment causing bacterial infection and a build-up of gas which
may constrict the lungs. It is essential to allow the tortoise to
drink right up until hibernation in order to avoid dehydration.

> **Tip** A warm bath will usually stimulate defecation. So I bath mine twice a week until they do not produce anything for 2 consecutive baths

NB.

Tortoises that are usually allowed to roam in the garden should
not be permitted to do this once feeding has been stopped,
otherwise they may eat plant material from the garden.

Do you worm the tortoise prior to hibernation?

Again you want a 'yes'. Ideally this should be done a couple of months before the tortoise goes into hibernation. The reason for doing it then is that otherwise the worms might take the opportunity of a depressed immune system during the hibernation to multiply and so, when the tortoise wakes, it may have a heavy burden.

How do you ensure adequate bodyweight prior to hibernation?

The tortoise should be weighed and measured to see if it has attained enough weight for its size. There are several methods of assessing weight to length ratio but perhaps the most well known is the Jackson Ratio (Fig. 1.9).

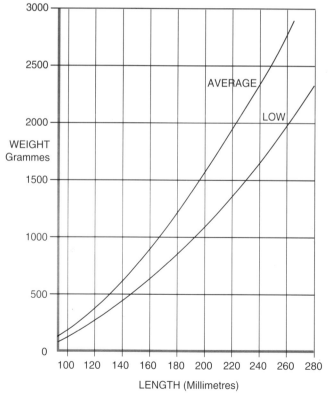

Fig. 1.9 The Jackson Ratio. Reproduced by kind permission of the British Chelonia Group

It must be remembered that this applies to Hermans and Spur-thighed tortoises only.

Describe the hibernation accommodation and siting in detail.

There are two main accommodation techniques.

1   Box method –

    a   Put the tortoise into a ventilated container just a little bigger than itself.

    b   Line the box with shredded paper and then pack more around the tortoise.

> **Tip** Avoid straw and hay if possible as they may contain fungal spores

    c   Place the container inside a larger ventilated container and pack the spaces between the two with an insulation material, e.g. polystyrene, vermiculite, newspaper, shredded paper.

    d   Ensure the small container is tortoise-proof and the larger container is both predator- and escape-proof.

    e   Place the boxes somewhere dry and weatherproof where the temperature will remain between 0 and 10°C. (Any colder and the tortoise may suffer from frost bite, any hotter and it may wake up.)

2   Fridge method – (my preference)

    a   Place the tortoise in a small, stout, ventilated container with some packing for comfort.

    b   Put the container in a **ventilated** fridge (not one that is used for storing food!) that has been set (and tested) to run at 4–6°C.

    c   Place the fridge somewhere dry and weatherproof.

Whichever method is used care must be taken when deciding where to leave the container/fridge because, for example, if it is left in a garage there is the possibility of carbon monoxide poisoning.

How often do you check the tortoise during hibernation?
If the tortoise is hibernating properly careful checks will not disturb it. These are necessary for the following reasons:

> Tip Placing a min/max thermometer inside the tortoise's container allows accurate monitoring

- Temperature monitoring.
- Monitoring weight loss. An adult tortoise should lose approximately 1% of its body weight each month. If it is losing too much it may need to be woken up.

If it should wake up it is advisable to keep it awake rather than let it re-hibernate as it may not have the resources to wake up properly for a second time.

At the end of hibernation do you wake the tortoise up yourself or allow it to wake up on its own?
Either is acceptable depending on circumstances. In the wild the Mediterranean tortoise will hibernate for approximately 3–4 months, rousing itself when the temperature begins to warm up and many owners allow this natural pattern to prevail. However, the owner may wish to control the length of hibernation for a number of reasons:

1   The tortoise is small or young.
2   The tortoise is not heavy enough to survive a full length hibernation.
3   Personal convenience. If the owners are going to be away at about the time the tortoise usually comes out of hibernation, they may not want to leave it with someone who is not sure what to do.

4   The tortoise has been hibernating for too long. (If it is still in hibernation after 5 months it should be woken.)

If it wakes up by itself, how do you know when it has done so?
Hopefully the answer will be that, once the temperature starts to warm up, daily checks are made.

Please describe what you do immediately the tortoise has woken up and for the following few days.
Post-hibernation procedure should be something akin to the following:

1   Once awake (or to induce arousal) bring the container into a warm room for a few hours.
2   Remove the tortoise from the box into a warm, bright environment
3   When **fully** awake place in a warmish bath just deep enough for it to drink properly. This is for two main reasons:
    a   Re-hydration is very important
    b   Bathing will encourage urination, thus eliminating the toxic by-products of metabolism (uric acid) that have built up during hibernation
        Some people like to put glucose in the water. This is only necessary if the tortoise has used up too much fat and the liver has started breaking down the stored sugars.
4   Check the tortoise carefully for any indications of ill health
5   Food can be offered when it is fully awake and up to normal temperatures (usually the next day). The first feed should be a small one to allow the digestive system to become accustomed to receiving food again. If the tortoise is not eating after four or five days there is probably something wrong.

HISTORY

TERRAPINS

ANIMAL'S DETAILS

Name _____

Species _____

Sex _____

Where did you get it from? _____

Approximate age _____

How long have you had it? _____

When and with what was it last wormed? _____

HOUSING

Please fill in the relevant section (inside/outside). If the
terrapin is housed both outside and inside at different times of
the year fill in both sections and specify when each is
applicable.

OUTSIDE

Describe the accommodation, including measurements and
depth of the pond and the whole enclosure _____

_____

_____

_____

_____

_____

_____

_____

_____

_____

Does the terrapin overwinter in the pond? _____

If so, how deep is the mud at the bottom? _____

INSIDE

Describe the set-up, including measurements of the overall accommodation and the water area.

_____

_____

_____

_____

_____

_____

_____

_____

Describe the access from the water to the land area _____

_____

_____

What is the substrate on the land area? _____

LIGHTING

Is there any UV provision? (State type of tube used and how frequently it is changed) _____

How high above the substrate/water is the UV positioned? _____

Is there a spotlight/basking light? (State type and wattage) _____

For how long are the lights on each day? _____

HEATING

What is the temperature of the water? _____

How is this maintained? (State type of heater, if used) _____

_____

What type of thermometer is used to monitor the water temperature? _____

Does the water heater have a guard around it? _____

Is it connected to a thermostat? _____

What is the background temperature in the
accommodation? _____

How is this maintained? (State type of heater if used) _____
_____

Does the background heater have a guard around it? _____

Is it connected to a thermostat? _____

Do you use a min./max. thermometer in the
accommodation? _____

What is the temperature under the spotlight/basking light? _____

WATER

This applies to both inside and outside accommodation

What type of (and capacity) filter is used? _____

How often is the water changed – partially? _____

totally? _____

Describe the process for changing the water _____
_____

Is the pond natural and self-sustaining? _____

FEEDING

How often is the terrapin fed? _____

List **all** food items given, including quantity and frequency, *or*
complete a diet sheet. **See Appendix I** _____

_____

_____

_____

_____

_____

_____

_____

What supplements are provided and how often? _____

How do you ensure the supplement is delivered? _____

_____

What are the insects fed on? _____

Describe the method of feeding (e.g. throw food into the water,

hand-fed) _____

SOCIAL GROUPING

How many other terrapins share the accommodation?

Male _____

Female _____

Are they all the same species? _____

ANY OTHER COMMENTS

_____

_____

_____

_____

_____

_____

_____

EXPLANATION OF QUESTIONS
TERRAPINS

[WHERE A SPECIFIC QUESTION IS NOT EXPLAINED, REFER *TO THE SNAKES AND LIZARDS SECTION*]

HOUSING

Some people keep their terrapins in indoor housing all year round, some in an outside enclosure all year, and others keep them in inside accommodation during the winter and outside during the summer. It is important to establish which of these is relevant and to get as much detail as possible about each type of accommodation.

OUTSIDE
Describe the accommodation, including measurements and depth of the pond and the whole enclosure.
Ideally this should be as large as possible (obviously the more individuals housed the larger it should be) and include a land area as well as a pond. Specific points to check are:

1   (As a general guideline) the water depth for adult animals is approximately 1½–2½ times the length of the terrapin.

Tip For an adult this usually equates to 45–75 cm

(For hatchlings and juveniles see Tip box in inside accommodation section.)
2   The height of the enclosing fence or wall is enough to deter, for example, unauthorised children.

3   The surrounding fence or wall extends into the ground at least 6 inches (15 cm) as terrapins will often dig their way out, given the chance.

4   The area is exposed to the sun for most of the day.

5   There is shade/cover provided.

6   There is easy access into and out of the pond.

7   In the wild, terrapins can often be seen basking in the sun on, for example, a log, over the surface of the pond. They are then able to launch themselves into the water if they become alarmed. A similar set up in captivity is a very good idea.

Does the terrapin overwinter in the pond?

So many terrapins are being dumped that it is not unusual for rescue centres to have a very large collection and to let them live as naturally as possible in an outside pond all year round. It is not as common with private owners because, for a large portion of the year, the owner has no contact with the terrapin. Either method is acceptable but if they are overwintered there are certain criteria that should be adhered to, or losses may occur:

1   The water should be at least 2½ feet (75 cm) deep

2   There should be mud at the bottom at least 6 inches (15 cm) deep. This enables the terrapins to be completely covered (protected) during their hibernation

3   The surface area of the pond should be greater than the depth in order to avoid oxygen deficiency

4   Individuals of less than 4 inches (10 cm) long should not be over-wintered

5   The terrapin should be in good health

If so, how deep is the mud at the bottom?

– See above

INSIDE

Describe the set-up including measurements of the overall accommodation and the water area.

Like the outside set-up, this should be as large as possible, and the more individuals it contains the larger it should be. You need to check that:

- there is a discrete land area, not just a rock or two protruding above the surface. This not only provides opportunity for environmental enrichment but provides a safe area for sunbathing which, as already mentioned, is an activity that is very much enjoyed in the wild.

> Tip Regular sunbathing helps to prevent fungal infections affecting the shell

- the spotlight/basking light is placed over the land area. This encourages the terrapin to come out of the water regularly
- any glass in the vivarium is toughened. (I discovered to my cost that ordinary glass will be broken with exasperating regularity. The novelty of walking into the reptile room and discovering the terrapins paddling about on a soaking floor quickly wore off when it happened twice in two months.)
- the water is of sufficient depth and size to allow natural swimming behaviour.

> Tip Hatchlings should have about 5 cm of water and juveniles approx. the width of the shell. Adults need approx. 1½–2½ times the length of the shell

Describe the access from the water to the land area.

Whilst terrapins are surprisingly agile, a gradual slope that makes access between land and water is preferable, as the easier it is the more readily they will use it. A simple wooden ramp that extends under water will suffice.

What is the substrate on the land area?

Almost anything will do, as long as it does not matter if it gets wet. However, depending on the size of the land area, something like 'astro turf' is invaluable as it does not get dragged into the water as does, for example, peat or bark, and it is easily cleaned and disinfected.

> Tip It is also a good idea to provide an egg-laying site (sand or peat) for a female to lay eggs. (See relevant section in Lizard history

LIGHTING

Is there a spotlight/basking light?

This should be placed over the land area, and the temperature (at terrapin level) should reach approximately 32°C.

For how long are the lights on each day?

For terrapins kept inside, a winter cooling down is not necessary unless you want them to breed. Therefore, the lighting cycle can remain constant year round. The length of time the lights are on is not critical; I recommend about 10–12 hours a day.

> Tip I can think of no conceivable reason why anyone should want to breed red-ears when there are so many in rescue centres in need of a home.

HEATING

What is the temperature of the water?

Ideally, 24–26°C during the daytime and about 20°C at night, although I know of several examples of terrapins kept successfully in water colder than this.

How is this maintained?

If the room is heated it may not be necessary to provide additional heating for the water. If heating is required the most common method is to use adjustable aquarium heaters. These come in various sizes and, if the water area is very large, it may be necessary to use more than one.

What type of thermometer is used to monitor the water temperature?

The strips that stick onto the outside of the glass are commonly used. The problem with these thermometers is that they can be affected by the ambient temperature outside the tank and I have found that they are not especially reliable or accurate. However, any thermometer that is left in the water runs the risk of being smashed by the terrapin. Therefore, if using the stick-on strip type, I would advise regular double-checking by placing an ordinary thermometer in the water for a minute or two and, if a water thermometer is used, it should have a fixed guard around it.

> **Tip** The problem with aquarium thermometers is that they only register the current temperature. This is probably not a problem if using a heater in the water, but if you are relying on the general room temperature to maintain the water temperature there is no way of knowing what it is at, say, 2.00 am (unless you want to get up and test it). The only way of getting an approximate reading is by having a min./max. thermometer in the accommodation and working out what the water temperature is at any given time in relation to the temperature in the accommodation.

Does the water heater have a guard around it?

As with thermometers, if using a heater that stays in the water, it will almost certainly get broken unless it has a fixed guard around it.

Is it connected to a thermostat?

Most aquarium heaters have an in-built thermostat. Obviously, it is just as important to regulate the temperature of the terrapins' water as it is for any other reptile environment.

What is the temperature under the spotlight/basking light?

See under 'lighting'

WATER

Water quality is a very important issue. Dirty water is one of the major causes of disease in terrapins.

What type of (and capacity) filter is used?

In almost every instance a filter is essential. There are three basic types of filter available:

1 Under-gravel – This is not suitable for terrapins, as it cannot cope with the amount of debris generated.
2 Internal canister – The main problem with this type is that because it is sited in the water it takes up space that would otherwise be swimming space. In a large outside enclosure this may not be a problem, but in an inside vivarium it invariably is.
3 External canister – This is the type of choice for indoor accommodation as there is no restriction on size.

The filter capacity should be as large as possible as terrapins generate a tremendous amount of debris. The capacity of a filter is governed by how much water it can filter per hour. For fish tanks it is recommended that the entire water content is filtered each hour. *However*, for terrapins the filter needs to deal with 2–2½ times the total water content per hour.

> **Tip** The formula for calculating how much water is contained in a large tank/pond etc. is length × width × depth (in feet) × 6.24 = total capacity in gallons

How often is the water changed?

Even with a powerful filter the water will become dirty. Partial water changes will reduce this but a complete change of water should be carried out regularly.

Obviously, the frequency of each will depend on:

- the size of the water area
- how many terrapins are housed together
- whether food is left in the water (see feeding section)

However, to give you a rough guideline: a water area of approximately bath size and 1½ feet deep (45 cm), housing 2 terrapins that are not fed in the same tank, will probably need both a partial and a total water change weekly.

Describe the process for changing the water.
You need to consider:

- the simplicity (or otherwise) of the process
- whether the water can be drained away completely.

The more difficult the process, the less likely it is to be carried out regularly or efficiently.

Is the pond natural and self-sustaining?
Some people, particularly rescue centres or those with a large number of terrapins, will keep them in an outside pond all year round. If this is a large, natural type of pond it may be that it does not require filters or water changes as the vegetation will take care of the cleaning process naturally.

However, if the terrapin is brought in with a problem that relates to dirty water then it may be that the pond is not as self-correcting as they had thought, or that it cannot cope with the number of terrapins in it.

FEEDING

How often is the terrapin fed?
As with the lizards, how often is related to how much. Whilst daily feeding will help with environmental enrichment, many people prefer not to feed on a daily basis but maybe 3 × weekly. Common sense must be employed: if the animal appears to be putting on weight then a reduction in the amount of food is necessary.

List all food items given, including quantity and frequency.

It would be preferable if the client completes a diet sheet as this will make it easier to assess the overall diet. Terrapins are omnivorous, glutinous, unfussy and the most messy of creatures in their feeding habits. Listed below are some of their more favoured foods.

Fish – e.g. whitebait, sprats. It is better to feed whole, small fish rather than chopped up larger ones, but not essential. If too much fish that has been previously frozen is given it may lead to a thiamine deficiency. (This is because fish that have been frozen contain thiaminase which destroys thiamine.)

Prawns – These are **extremely addictive** and should not be given too often or in large quantities.

River shrimp – These can be given live and provide a good source of environmental enrichment.

Meat – This should be given in the natural form, that is, mice, **not** cat or dog food because the latter is too high in protein and, if given over a prolonged period, may result in kidney and liver damage. (This applies to **all** reptiles) Some people advocate cat or dog food if it is used sparingly because it is convenient and not as off-putting as having to deal with dead mice. I feel that if you give someone 'licence' to use it there is the possibility they will abuse it.

Whole adult mice should be chopped up into 'gulp sized' pieces; pinkies (baby mice) can usually be fed whole.

Snails – It is preferable not to use the ordinary 'garden' variety as they may carry parasites that could infect the terrapin. Giant African land snails are commonly available from reptile shops and should lessen the risk of parasite contamination. They can be obtained at whatever size is suitable for the terrapin to eat in one gulp.

Crickets/locusts

Fruit/Vegetables – Particular favourites are watercress, banana and dandelion leaves, but they will take almost anything and individual animals will show their own preferences.

Pelleted food – e.g. Reptomin pellets. These are often sold as a 'complete diet' but should be used as part of a varied one.

Freeze-dried food – As the name implies, this consists of various water creatures, such as daphnia and shrimps, that have been freeze dried. Again, these are not to be used as a complete diet. As with other reptiles variety is the key to a good diet.

Terrapins are voracious hunters, and individuals that live outside may also supplement their diet with any natural fauna and flora that happens to come along, for example pond weed, tadpoles, frogs, newts, fish, water invertebrates, etc. (or anything that looks like it might be edible, e.g. duckling legs).

What supplements are provided and how often?

Terrapins do need additional supplementation (see Snakes & lizards section for further information).

How do you ensure the supplement is delivered?

Terrapins will only feed in water so there is a distinct possibility that if a powdered supplement is used it will be washed off in the water. One way around this is to give some or all of their food by hand. (When I say 'by hand' I do not mean with your fingers or you will probably lose them. Use plastic tweezers.) When the terrapin grabs the food it will usually take the tweezers as well so plastic ones will reduce the possibility of damaging the mouth.

Another advantage of hand-feeding is that you are able to monitor each individual, ensuring that not only are they all eating but that they are each getting their fair share.

Describe the method of feeding.

The reason for this question may, in part, be ascertained by the above question, that is ensuring that each terrapin is eating sufficient food. However, it also has a bearing on the water quality. If food is thrown into the water and the terrapin/s are then left to their own devices it is certain that some of it will not be found and will therefore rot in the water. This will necessitate more frequent water changes.

Some people feed the terrapin in a separate container (a large plastic box will suffice) and this will make a big difference in keeping the water cleaner.

SOCIAL GROUPING

How many other terrapins share the accommodation?

There is not generally a problem with multiple males being housed together but it might become a problem if the females are vastly outnumbered as they may be constantly harassed by the males at certain times of the year.

Sexing immature red-ears is very difficult but sexing mature ones is very easy, the males having much longer front claws than the females.

Are they all the same species?

This may or may not be relevant, depending on the species. For example a snapping turtle is an absolute menace if mixed with anything else.

HISTORY

AMPHIBIANS

ANIMAL'S DETAILS

Name _____

Species _____

Sex _____

Where did you get it from? _____

Approximate age _____

How long have you had it? _____

HOUSING

VIVARIUM

What is the vivarium made of? _____

What are its measurements? _____

How is ventilation provided? _____

Where is the vivarium sited? _____

LIGHTING

What type of lighting is provided? _____

What wattage is it? _____

How high above the highest surface is it? _____

Does it have a guard around it? _____

For how long are the lights on each day? _____

HEATING

What is the temperature of the water? _____

How is this maintained? (State type of heater, if used) _____

_____

What type of thermometer is used to monitor the water temperature? _____

_____

Does the water heater have a guard around it? _____

Is it connected to a thermostat? _____

What is the background temperature in the accommodation?

   Day _____

   Night _____

How is this maintained? (State type of heater, if used) _____

_____

Does the background heater have a guard around it? _____

_____

Is it connected to a thermostat? _____

Do you use a min./max. thermometer in the accommodation? __

_____

What is the temperature under the spotlight? _____

HUMIDITY

What is the humidity? _____

Is there a humidity gauge? _____

DÉCOR – LAND

What proportion of the vivarium is land area? _____

What substrate is used? _____

How deep is the substrate? _____

How is the humidity/dampness maintained? _____

Describe the land area. (Include items of furniture and method of access from the water) _____

_____

_____

Are there any plants? (Specify whether real or plastic) _____

_____

If real, what species are they? _____

Have they been re-potted into soil? _____

Is a spotlight/basking light provided? (Give details) _____

How frequently is the vivarium cleaned out? _____

What cleaning solution is used? _____

DÉCOR – WATER

How large is the water area? _____

How deep is the water? _____

What substrate is used? _____

What other items of décor are there? (e.g. logs, rocks,

drainpipes) _____

_____

_____

Is there a water filter? (If yes, state type [undergravel, internal,

external] and capacity) _____

How is the water dechlorinated? _____

How often is the water changed? _____

FEEDING

List **all** food items fed and how often each is given _____

_____

_____

_____

_____

_____

How often is the animal fed? _____

What supplements are provided and how often? _____

If feeding with insects, how do you ensure the supplement

is delivered? _____

_____

What are the insects fed on? _____

SOCIAL GROUPING

Does it live alone or with other individuals? (State species and numbers) _____

_____

What is the ratio of sexes, if known? _____

HANDLING

How frequently is it handled? _____

Describe how this is done _____

_____

_____

COOLING DOWN

Please describe fully the process of cooling down, length of cooling and warming back up. _____

_____

_____

_____

_____

_____

ANY OTHER COMMENTS

_____

_____

_____

_____

_____

_____

_____

EXPLANATION OF QUESTIONS
AMPHIBIANS

[WHERE A SPECIFIC QUESTION IS NOT EXPLAINED, REFER TO THE SNAKES & LIZARDS SECTION]

HOUSING

VIVARIUM

What is the vivarium made of?

The vast majority of amphibians will require water areas and high humidity. There are a small number that are entirely terrestrial but these too will need a fairly humid environment, therefore, a wooden vivarium is not usually the best material. The most commonly used is glass or fibreglass, although these materials are not without their problems because:

- both provide little in the way of thermal insulation
- all-glass vivaria can make the animal feel rather exposed, being visible from all sides. The solution is to blank-off three sides with an opaque material, such as black paper taped to the outside or, even better, something that will provide some insulation as well, e.g. polystyrene.

What are its measurements?

The factors to be considered here are the same as those previously discussed in the Snakes & lizards section. It is particularly important to ascertain whether the animal is arboreal, e.g. White's Tree Frog.

How is ventilation provided?

Again, this has been discussed previously. Providing ventilation in an all-glass vivarium is not easy, and usually limited to

57

ensuring that the lid or part of it (depending on the size) is covered with an appropriately sized wire mesh. Good ventilation is especially important in humid situations.

Where is the vivarium sited?

It should be away from heaters, windows, draughts, or any other environment that would affect the carefully regulated temperature and have potentially fatal results.

LIGHTING
What type of lighting is provided?

There is some discussion as to whether UV lighting is necessary for amphibians. The first factors to take into consideration are whether they are nocturnal or diurnal and then, if diurnal, what type of habitat is natural. For example, if they inhabit thick vegetation it is unlikely that they receive much sunlight. Having said this, many people like to use a low-level UV, full spectrum light, such as the Reptisun 2.0, 'just in case' and/or for the improved aesthetic appearance resulting from enhanced colours.

> **Tip** If real plants are used, a full spectrum light is essential.

Some form of lighting is necessary, not only so that you can see into the vivarium but also so that the animal can regulate its day/night cycle. An incandescent light, or being in a well-lit room at the very least, is needed.

What wattage is it?

You need to consider the following points:

1   In a small vivarium a light bulb can generate a substantial increase in the temperature, which must be taken into consideration.

2   A high wattage light bulb can cause a hot spot that is too
     hot and may result in 'cooked frog'.

3   The higher the wattage the more intense the light. For
     species from densely vegetated areas this may be
     detrimental.

How high above the highest surface is it?

This question is asked for two reasons. First, if it is too low the
frog might be able to jump onto it and therefore burn itself and,
second, the lower it is the greater the hot spot created.

For how long are the lights on each day?

Unless cooling down, most amphibians respond well to a 12
hours on and 12 hours off cycle, preferably with a slow dimming
of the lights rather than a sudden on and off.

HEATING

Tip   As a general rule, European and temperate species do not require any additional heating,
       provided that the room they are kept in maintains temperatures similar to those of their
       native environment.

[See the section on terrapins for further explanation]

What is the temperature of the water?

This will very much depend on the species. If the
accommodation is heated then additional heating in the water
may not be necessary. However, this question is to ensure that
the owner is aware of the water temperature.

What is the background temperature in the accommodation?

Again, this will vary between species. European animals require
lower temperatures than tropical ones. As with all other species,
there should be a drop in temperature at night, usually of about 5°C.

How is this maintained?

Heating provision for amphibians is different from the reptiles previously discussed. (See Fig. 1.10)

- It is a very simple matter to 'cook' amphibians with over-enthusiastic heating.
- If an all glass/fibreglass vivarium is used there is an exception to the rule where heat mats are concerned. A mat should be placed on the **outside** of the walls or under the floor. However, a heat gradient is still necessary so the mat should not cover the entire wall or floor.

> **Tip** A deep layer of substrate or water will absorb the heat, significantly reducing the effectiveness.

- Other forms of heating must be used with extreme caution as they may overheat the vivarium.

> **Tip** Placing a sheet of polystyrene on the back of the heat mat will help to direct the heat in the desired direction and not into the room.

Is it connected to a thermostat?

Heat mats should be connected to specialised 'mat stats'. These are not as precise as other forms of thermostat and so

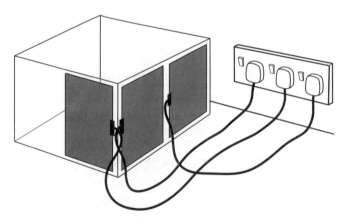

Fig. 1.10 Diagram showing the use of heat mats.

you may need to do some fiddling around to work out the exact temperatures, but they are designed specifically for heat mats. One thing to bear in mind with this form of heating is that during a cold spell they may not be sufficient to maintain required temperatures if the ambient room temperature falls too low.

What is the temperature under the spotlight?

Some diurnal species may require a hot spot but it may be detrimental to others. It is therefore important to know which category a particular species falls into and what the required temperature should be.

HUMIDITY
What is the humidity?

With many species this is surprisingly low. Provided there is an adequate water area, the general humidity may be as low as 50–60%. Care should be taken to ensure the land area substrate does not dry out.

DÉCOR – LAND
What proportion of the vivarium is land area?

This should vary depending on whether the species is:

- totally/predominantly aquatic, e.g. African clawed toad, axolotl (Fig. 1.11)
- semi-aquatic, e.g. most of the commonly kept amphibians (Fig. 1.12)
- totally/predominantly terrestrial or arboreal, e.g. tree frogs, mole salamanders (Fig. 1.13)

In addition, within each of these categories (particularly the semi-aquatic), the requirements may vary between species.

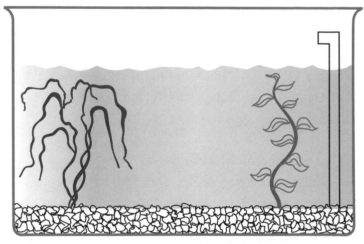

Fig. 1.11 Totally/predominantly aquatic species

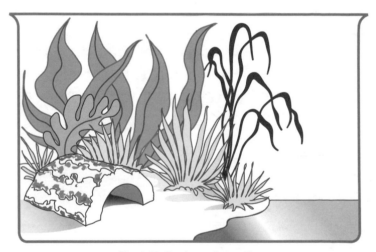

Fig. 1.12 Semi-aquatic species

What substrate is used?

Amphibians are extremely sensitive to chemicals and this must be remembered when selecting a suitable substrate, something like peat for example should be avoided so too bark chippings. I prefer to use moss from a reptile shop as this has been sterilised.

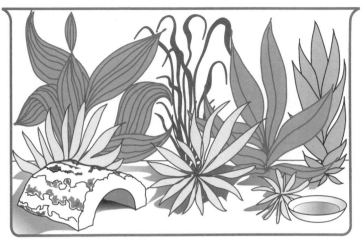

Fig. 1.13 Totally/predominantly terrestrial species

Gravel (again from the reptile/aquarist shop), whilst not presenting any dangers from hidden chemicals can cause a problem if ingested with the food. If this is used it should be of a size that will not be readily eaten along with the food item.

How deep is the substrate?
Species that like to burrow into the ground, such as horned frogs, need a deeper layer than, say, tree frogs.

Describe the land area –

• Most species will require areas in which to hide and this can be in the form of plants, rocks, branches, cork bark, and so on. For arboreal species, plenty of branches using the full height of the vivarium should be used, together with hides at various heights.
• Specialist reptile or aquarist shops have a large range of items of décor available. If using bits and pieces from the garden they must be thoroughly disinfected and then rinsed until there is **no trace** of the disinfectant left.

63

- Although décor is required in the land area, it should not be too cluttered as this will make observation and cleaning difficult.
- There should be easy access from the water to the land area. It must be remembered that **frogs drown!** There should also be rocks in the water for them to climb out onto.

Are there any plants?

Rainforest species in particular may need plants to simulate the natural environment.

If real, what species are they?

Apart from the obvious reason that they may be toxic, they need to be of sufficient strength to bear the weight of the animal. Species such as the cheese plant, mother-in-law's tongue, philodendrons and some of the sturdier ficus are often used.

> **Tip** Regular removal of dead leaves and general plant maintenance will reduce the risk of bacteria and mould building up in the vivarium.

Have they been re-potted into soil?

The compost that nurseries use will probably contain pesticides or fertilisers, which can be toxic to the animal. Take as much of the original compost as possible away from the roots and re-pot the whole plant into clean topsoil.

Is a spotlight/basking light provided?

See heating section

How frequently is the vivarium cleaned out?

All frogs and toads secrete a chemical (of varying toxicity). This will build up in the environment and, whilst it may not be toxic to humans, it will reach levels that may harm the animal itself.

- Regular cleaning of **all** areas and items in the vivarium is essential. This should be done every 2 or 3 days by spraying down the sides of the vivarium, all items of furniture (rocks, plants, branches, etc.) and spraying, washing or changing the substrate, depending on what is being used.

- The water used to spray clean the environment should be hot and dechlorinated. (Do not spray hot water on real plants or the amphibians!)
- Potted plants should have the top layer of soil replenished every couple of months or so.
- A regular, thorough cleaning should also be carried out. The frequency will depend on the size of the vivarium and the number of animals housed, but should be done at least monthly.
- During total clean-outs the animals should be removed to a separate container.

What cleaning solution is used?

- **All amphibians are extremely sensitive to chemicals.**
- As a rule the only solution used should be hot water.
- It is important to remember that any water used in the vivarium should be dechlorinated. In some areas, allowing water to stand for 2 or 3 days or so before use may be sufficient to remove all traces of chlorine. Find out what other amphibian keepers in the area do but if in doubt use a dechlorinating solution. Dechlorinator can be obtained at most reptile and aquarist shops.
- If a disinfectant has to be used it must be thoroughly rinsed off so that no trace of it remains.

DÉCOR – WATER
How large is the water area?
Some species require more water than others. The minimum, for those that do not require a large area, it that it must be large enough for them to be able to sit comfortably.

How deep is the water?

Again, this depends on the species but, as I have already said and cannot emphasise enough, **frogs drown**. Therefore, for the predominantly terrestrial and semi-aquatic species it is a good idea not to make the water area too deep.

What substrate is used?

It is not a necessity to use a substrate in the water area, indeed, if it is only a small bowl it is not practical. Any that is used will have the disadvantage of trapping waste and making cleaning that much more difficult.

If a substrate is used it is usually gravel or, preferably, stones. It should be large enough to ensure that the animal will not accidentally ingest it and, ideally, obtained from a reptile or aquarist shop, because garden gravel especially can contain all sorts of contaminants.

What other items of décor are there?

The two main purposes of these items are to provide:

- places to hide (e.g. drainpipes, logs, floating plants, etc.)
- areas where the animal can escape the water (e.g. rocks around the edges and/or in the middle)

A sloping slate (see Fig. 1.14) is ideal as it covers both points.

> **Tip** The formula for calculating how much water is contained in a *small* tank is:
> Metric – length × width × depth (cm's) ÷ 1000 = total capacity in litres
> Imperial – length × width × depth (inches) ÷ 280 = total capacity in gallons

Is there a water filter?

Obviously, this will depend on the size of the water area. If a filter is used the same principles apply for amphibians as previously discussed for terrapins.

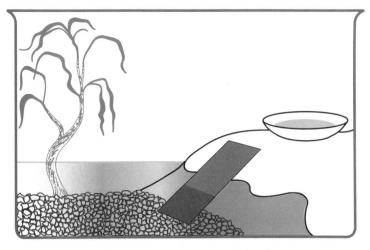

Fig. 1.14 Diagram showing sloping slate

Totally or predominantly aquatic set-ups should have some kind of aeration. The filter will usually serve this purpose, particularly if the returning water pipe is sited on or just above the surface. If there is no filter an aquarium aerator should be used.

How is the water dechlorinated?

There are two main methods for removing the chlorine from the water, depending on the chlorine levels in your area:

1 Allow the water to stand for at least 48 hours, preferably longer.
2 The use of dechlorinating solution. This involves adding a small amount of chemical to a specified quantity of water.

[*See the earlier section on cleaning solutions for further details*.] The alternative is to use clean rainwater.

It is important to remember that **all** water with which the amphibian might come into contact (that used for spraying, cleaning, handling, or in temporary containers whilst cleaning out) should be treated in this way first.

How often is the water changed?

This will depend on a number of factors such as:

- whether a filter is used
- the size of the water area
- how many individuals are housed together

Many species will defaecate in the water but they also use it to rehydrate so it is important to keep it clean. Small containers or bowls should be changed daily, larger areas (depending on the above factors) should have **at least** a partial water change weekly and a total change every 2–3 weeks.

FEEDING

As a rule amphibians tend to be insectivorous, eating land and waterborne insects and larvae. Some will also take small fish and frogs.

In captivity their diet usually revolves around crickets as the staple item with a variety of other items given once or twice a week, e.g. waxworms, flies, locusts, small fish, pinkies.

SOCIAL GROUPING

Does it live alone or with other individuals?

Many species of amphibian will benefit from company, particularly frogs and toads. Indeed for some, if breeding is desired, it is essential as competition will stimulate the process, for example in fire-bellied toads. For others though, such as the horned frog, it can be fatal.

Vivariums should not hold mixed amphibian species as the toxins secreted by one species may be harmful to another.

Tip With frogs and toads one method that may help is to notice which ones tend to be more vocal; these are probably male.

What is the ratio of sexes?

For most species there does not have to be an even mix of males and females, but common sense dictates that if there are say five or six males and one female this is not an ideal ratio. Very often, however, this will not be known as it can be difficult to sex amphibians.

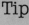 **Tip** Another method is to watch them when mating. A male will grasp the female around the waist and stay there, often for several hours or even days. If a male grabs another male by mistake, he should let go fairly soon.

HANDLING

How frequently is it handled?

Most amphibians do not appreciate being handled and so this should be kept to a minimum. Although one species that does not seem to object too violently is the White's tree frog.

Describe how this is done.

Chemicals on our hands, whether sweat or hand cream, will be absorbed by the animal's skin, so it is not a matter of just picking them up carefully. One of the following procedures must be observed:

1   Ideally, plastic or surgical gloves should be worn (non-powdered) and then rinsed in dechlorinated water and left wet.
2   If no gloves are available then hands should be washed in hot water (no soap) and then rinsed in dechlorinated water and left wet.

COOLING DOWN

- Many amphibians experience a natural cool season in the wild, but many do not so it is important to establish in which category a particular species belongs.

- Different species have different requirements for a cooling down, such as the minimum temperature, so specific research is necessary.
- Many species do have a cool season in the wild but it is not necessary to duplicate this in captivity unless breeding is required. So, although it is beneficial to allow the animal to follow its natural life cycle, it may not be essential.

2 SAMPLE COMPLETED FORMS

These are real life examples that have been completed in order to illustrate correct husbandry methods.

I have tried to include a wide variety of approaches so that you can be aware of as many as possible. However, it is not exhaustive and you may well come across other equally acceptable methods.

The species covered are those most commonly kept but again, it is by no means complete.

HISTORY

SNAKES & LIZARDS – CORN SNAKE

ANIMAL'S DETAILS

Name _____ **Kellogg**

Species (and subspecies if known) _____ **Corn snake /**

Elaphe guttata

Sex _____ **Male**

Where did you get it from? _____ **Breeder**

Approximate age _____ **3 years**

(av. life span 15–20 years)

How long have you had it? _____ **2 ½ years**

When and with what was it last wormed? _____ **4 months**

ago with Panacur 10% soln

HOUSING

VIVARIUM

What is the vivarium made of? _____ **Wood & glass**

What are the measurements? _____ **6′l × 2′h × 18″ d**

(183 × 61 × 46 cm)

How is ventilation provided? _____ **A vent at either**

end, 1 high up & 1 low

down, each approx.

8″ × 4″ (20 × 10 cm)

LIGHTING

Is there any UV provision? (State type of tube used and how
frequently it is changed) _____ **No**

How high above the substrate is the UV positioned?_____ **N/A**

Is there a spotlight/basking light? (State
type & wattage) _____ **100w spot**
Does the spotlight/basking light have a guard around it? ___ **Yes**
For how long are the lights on each day?

Summer _____ **Approx. 14 hrs**

Winter _____ **Approx. 9 hrs when not hibernating**

HEATING

What type of heater is used? _____ **Tubular greenhouse heater**
Does it have a guard around it? _____ **Yes**
Is it connected to a thermostat? _____ **Yes**
State the background temperatures: Summer   Winter

	Summer	Winter
Day	**25–30°C**	**18°C (hibernation)**
Night	**22–25°C**	**18°C (hibernation)**

Do you use min./max. thermometers? _____ **Yes**
What is the temperature under the
spotlight/basking light? _____ **32°C**
Is all the heating and lighting equipment at the
same end of the vivarium? _____ **Yes**
What is the temperature difference between the
'hot end' and the 'cool end'? _____ **Approx. 5°C**

HUMIDITY

What is the humidity? _____ **40–50%**
Is there a humidity gauge? _____ **Yes**
How is it provided? ____ **Large container filled with damp peat**

DÉCOR

What substrate is used? _____ **Proprietary beech chips**
How deep is the substrate? _____ **Approx. 2″ (5 cm)**
How frequently is the vivarium cleaned out? ____ **Spot cleaning
daily, total clean out as necessary
usually approx. every 5–6 months**

What cleaning solution is used? _____ **Tamodine-E**

Describe the hide box/es _____ **Cork bark, shredded paper and rock pile**

Is there a covered, damp moss/peat container? _____ **Yes**

What other items of décor are there?

(rocks, branches, drain pipes, plastic

or real plants, etc,) _____ **Mopani wood, thick branches**

FEEDING

List **all** food items given including quantity

and frequency *or* complete a diet sheet

(if fruit & vegetables list each type) _____ **1 or 2 mice weekly**

How often is the animal fed? _____ **Weekly**

What supplements are provided and how often? _____ **None**

If feeding with insects, how do you ensure the supplement is

delivered?

_____ **N/A**

What are the insects fed on? _____ **N/A**

What size is the water container? _____ **Bowl about 8″ across and 4″ deep** (20 × 10 cm)

SOCIAL GROUPING

What other individuals of the same or different species share the

accommodation? _____ **Cornsnake**

How many are there of each and of what sex? _____ **1 × female**

Do they tend to mix with or ignore

each other? _____ **Often curled up together**

Is there at least one hide per individual? _____ **3**

COOLING DOWN

Please describe this process as fully as possible giving details on

when, for how long, heating, lighting, feeding, disturbance etc.

Cooling down starts Oct/Nov by gradually reducing the heating by 2°C per week until 18°C is reached day and night. Lighting time is also gradually reduced and the wattage of the spotlight changed to 60, then 40, and then turned off completely. When 18°C is achieved all lighting is turned off and the snakes are left undisturbed apart from changing the water and occasionally checking to make sure they are alright. Throughout the whole of the cooling down, feeding is suspended but water is still available. The process is then reversed, usually in Feb/March

ANY OTHER COMMENTS

_____

_____

_____

_____

_____

_____

_____

_____

ROSEWARNE
LEARNING CENTRE

HISTORY

SNAKES & LIZARDS – ROYAL PYTHON

ANIMAL'S DETAILS

Name _____ **Monty**

Species (and subspecies if known) _____ **Royal Python /**
Python regius

Sex _____ **Male**

Where did you get it from? _____ **Friend**

Approximate age _____ **6 years** (av. life span 20–30 years)

How long have you had it? _____ **2 years**

When and with what was it last wormed? _____ **Panacur,**
5 months ago

HOUSING

VIVARIUM

What is the vivarium made of? _____ **Fibreglass inside**
a wood casing

What are the measurements of the
vivarium? _____ **5'l × 2'd × 2'h** (152 × 61 × 61 cm)

How is ventilation provided? _____ **6″ (15 cm) ventilation**
grills at opposite ends

LIGHTING

Is there any UV provision? (State type of tube used and how
frequently it is changed) _____ **No**

How high above the substrate is the UV positioned? _____ **N/A**

Is there a spotlight/basking light? (State type & wattage) __ **100w**
spotlight

Does the spotlight/basking light have a guard around it? ___ **Yes**

How long are the lights on each day?

Summer _____ **6.00am–8.00pm**

Winter _____ **60w spot: 6.00am–6.00pm**

HEATING

What type of heater is used? _____ **Overhead ceramic**

Does it have a guard around it? _____ **Yes**

Is it connected to a thermostat? _____ **Yes**

State the background temperatures:	Summer	Winter
Day _____	**27–32°C**	**25–28°C**
Night _____	**22–25°C**	**20–23°C**

Do you use min./max. thermometers? _____ **Yes**

What is the temperature under the spotlight/basking light? __ **35°C**

Is all the heating and lighting equipment at the same

end of the vivarium? _____ **Yes**

What is the temperature difference between the

'hot end' and the 'cool end'? _____ **3–5°C depending**

upon time of year & day or night

HUMIDITY

What is the humidity? _____ **60% dry season (summer),**

85% rainy season (winter)

Is there a humidity gauge? _____ **Yes**

How is humidity provided?_____ **Spraying with tepid water**

2–3 times daily

DÉCOR

What substrate is used? _____ **Chipped bark & compost**

How deep is the substrate? _____ **Approx. 2″** (5 cm)

How frequently is the vivarium

cleaned out? _____ **Spot cleaned as necessary,**

totally cleaned approx. every 3 months

What cleaning solution is used? _____ **Ark-Klens**

Describe the hide box/es _____ **Large, hollowed out**
log, cork bark

Is there a covered, damp moss/peat

container? _____ **Yes, moss**

What other items of décor are there? (rocks, branches, drain

pipes, plants – plastic/real etc.) _____ **Branches, plastic plants**

FEEDING

List **all** food items given including quantity and frequency

or complete a diet sheet (If fruit & vegetables list

each type) _____ **Two mice once a week during dry season**

How often is the animal fed? _____ **Weekly**

What supplements are provided and how often? _____ **None**

If feeding with insects, how do you ensure the

supplement is delivered?_____ **N/A**

What are the insects fed on? _____ **N/A**

What size is the water container? _____ **Large washing up bowl**

SOCIAL GROUPING

What other individuals of the same or different

species share the accommodation? _____ **Royal python**

How many are there of each and of what sex _____ **1 × female**

Do they tend to mix with or ignore

each other? _____ **Often curl up together, other**
times ignore each other

Is there at least one hide per individual? _____ **Three in total**

COOLING DOWN

Please describe this process as fully as possible giving details on
when, for how long, heating, lighting, feeding, disturbances etc.

They don't get cooled down as such, but the temperatures are dropped slightly to 25–28°C during the day & 20–23°C at night during a simulated rainy season and the humidity is increased to 85% by spraying with warm water three or four times daily. Their 'rainy season' lasts for about 2 months during October & November.

ANY OTHER COMMENTS

_____

_____

_____

_____

_____

_____

_____

_____

_____

_____

HISTORY

SNAKES & LIZARDS – LEOPARD GECKO

ANIMAL'S DETAILS

Name _____ **Savannah**

Species (and subspecies if known) _____ **Leopard gecko/**

Eublepharis macularius

Sex _____ **Female**

Where did you get it from? _____ **Friend**

Approximate age _____ **Unknown, adult**

when acquired (av. life span 15–20 yrs)

How long have you had it? _____ **5 years**

When and with what was it last wormed? _____ **4 mths ago**

Panacur 10% soln

HOUSING

VIVARIUM

What is the vivarium made of? _____ **Wood & glass**

What are the measurements? _____ **4′l × 2′h × 2′d**

(122 × 61 × 61 cm)

How is ventilation provided? _____ **1 vent at the side**

near the bottom, 1 on the

front at the other end

near the top. Each vent

approx. 6″ × 4″ (15 × 10 cm)

LIGHTING

Is there any UV provision? (State type of tube used and how

frequently it is changed) _____ **Full spectrum**

daylight tube changed annually

How high above the substrate is the
UV positioned? _____ **Top of vivarium**

Is there a spotlight/basking light? (State
type & wattage) _____ **60w spotlight**

Does the spotlight/basking light have a guard around it_____ **Yes**

How long are the lights on each day?

   Summer _____ **14hrs**

   Winter _____ **8 hrs when not being hibernated**

HEATING

What type of heater is used? _____ **Tubular greenhouse heater**

Does it have a guard around it? _____ **Yes**

Is it connected to a thermostat? _____ **Yes**

State the background temperatures: Summer Winter

   Day _____ **26–30°C 18°C (hibernation)**

   Night _____ **22–25°C 18°C (hibernation)**

Do you use min./max. thermometers? _____ **Yes**

What is the temperature under the spotlight/basking light? __ **35°C**

Is all the heating and lighting equipment at the
same end of the vivarium? _____ **Yes**

What is the temperature difference between the
'hot end' and the 'cool end'? _____ **Hot end: 30°C,**
                                             cool end: 26°C

HUMIDITY

What is the humidity? _____ **50%**

Is there a humidity gauge? _____ **Yes**

How is it provided? _____ **Normal room humidity**
                                           & damp moss container

DÉCOR

What substrate is used? _____ **Lizard litter**

How deep is the substrate? _____ **Approx. 2″ (5 cm)**

How frequently is the vivarium cleaned out? ____ **Spot-cleaned daily, total clean-out as necessary**

What cleaning solution is used? _____ **Trigene**

Describe the hide box/es _____ **Cork bark pieces, cave made of rock & slate, margarine tubs**

Is there a covered, damp moss/peat container? _____ **Yes**

What other items of décor are there? (rocks, branches, drain pipes, plastic or real plants, etc) _____ **Sand area, rocks,**

FEEDING

List **all** food items given including quantity and frequency *or* complete a diet sheet (If fruit & vegetables list each type) _____ **Crickets – 5 or 6, two or three times a week, waxworms – 3 once a fortnight, pinkie – once a month**

How often is the animal fed? _____ **3 times a week**

What supplements are provided and how often? _____ **Nutrobal at every feed**

If feeding with insects, how do you ensure the supplement is delivered? _____ **Crickets are dusted with it and gecko is hand-fed at least three at each meal time to ensure powder is ingested**

What are the insects fed on? _____ **Fish flakes & apple**

What size is the water container? _____ **Plastic, fake pond type, about 6″ long, 3″ wide and 1″ deep** (15 × 7.5 × 2.5 cm)

SOCIAL GROUPING

What other individuals of the same or different species share the accommodation? _____ **4 other leopard geckos**

How many are there of each and of what sex? _____ **1 × male, 4 × females in total**

Do they tend to mix with or ignore
each other? _____ **A bit of both**

Is there at least one hide per individual? _____ **Yes**

COOLING DOWN

Please describe this process as fully as possible giving details
on when, for how long, heating, lighting, feeding, disturbances
etc.

**Temperature and lighting are gradually reduced during
October until 18°C is reached day and night. Temperature is
maintained at 18°C and all lighting is turned off for 2 months,
then heating and lighting is gradually returned to normal.
Feeding is suspended during this time.**

ANY OTHER COMMENTS

_____

_____

_____

_____

_____

_____

_____

_____

_____

HISTORY

SNAKES & LIZARDS – IGUANA

ANIMAL'S DETAILS

Name _____ **Iggy**

Species (and subspecies if known) ____ **Iguana / Iguana iguana**

Sex _____ **Female**

Where did you get it from? _____ **Reptile shop**

Approximate age _____ **5 yrs** (av. life span 15 – 20 years)

How long have you had it? _____ **Nearly 5 yrs**

When and with what was it last wormed? __ **6 months ago with**

Panacur

HOUSING

VIVARIUM

What is the vivarium made of?__ **Built in – brick, wood & glass**

What are its measurements? _____ **7′H, 5′D, 10′L**

(2.1 × 1.5 × 3 m)

How is ventilation provided? _____ **Sliding vents 2′ × 1′**

(60 × 30 cm) at each end,

one top & one bottom and a smaller

ventilation grill above the doors

LIGHTING

Is there any UV provision?

(State type of tube used and

how frequently it is changed) _____ **Arcadia D3 lights,**

changed every year (even though

it should be every 6 mths there

doesn't seem to be a problem)

How high above the substrate is the UV
positioned? _____ **Top of vivarium but next
to basking lamp**

Is there a spotlight/basking light?
(State type & wattage) _____ **Large reflector lamp 150w**

Does the spotlight/basking light have a guard around it ____ **Yes**

For how long are the lights on each day?

   Summer _____ **7am – 9 pm**

   Winter _____ **7am – 9pm**

HEATING

What type of heater is used?_ **4 × tubular greenhouse heaters**

Does it have a guard around it? _____ **Yes**

Is it connected to a thermostat? _____ **Yes**

State the background temperatures:

	Summer	Winter
Day _____	30°C	30°C
Night _____	25°C	25°C

Do you use min./max. thermometers? _____ **3 at various points**

What is the temperature under the spotlight/basking light? _ **35°C**

Is all the heating and lighting equipment
at the same end of the vivarium? _____ **Daylight/UV
tubes across whole ceiling,
spot & heaters at same end**

What is the temperature difference
between the hot end and the cool end? _____ **10°C**

HUMIDITY

What is the humidity? _____ **65–75%**

> **Tip** If keeping a male with 1 or more females, some keepers like to keep the humidity a little lower e.g. 40–45%. This is because high humidity stimulates breeding activity, which in turn may lead to a problem with aggression. Of course, there must be an adequate water container.

Is there a humidity gauge? _____ **Yes**

How is it provided? _____ **Automatic misting system**

DÉCOR

What substrate is used? __ **Potting compost & bark chippings**

How deep is the substrate? _____ **Approx. 2″ (5 cm) deep**

How frequently is the vivarium

cleaned out? _____ **Spot-cleaned daily**

What cleaning solution is used? _____ **Tamodine-E**

Describe the hide box/es ___ **Large cave made of rocks, large**
pieces of cork bark, clay drain pipes

Is there a covered, damp

moss/peat container? _____ **An area on the ground approx.**
18″ × 18″ (45 × 45 cm) containing damp
moss & substrate approx. 12″ (30 cm)
deep and surrounded by rocks

What other items of décor are there?

(rocks, branches, drain pipes, plastic or real

plants, etc,) _____ **Several branches, small pool, plastic plants**

FEEDING

List **all** food items given including quantity and

frequency *or* complete the diet sheet (if fruit &

vegetables list each type) _____ **A variety of fruit & veg.**
in rotation and when in season including:
broccoli, grated carrot, cauliflower, cabbage, runner beans &
leaves, curly kale, chard, spinach, watercress, chinese
leaves, mushrooms, tomatoes, cucumber, dandelion leaves &
flowers, groundsel, clover leaves & flowers, blackberries &
leaves, banana, apple, grapes, strawberries, melon, plum,
kiwi, peach, basil, coriander, rocket, iguana pellets

How often is the animal fed? _____ **Daily**

What supplements are provided and
how often? __ **Reptivite & a Ca-P supplement alternated daily**
If feeding with insects, how do you
ensure the supplement is delivered? _____ **N/A**
What are the insects fed on? _____ **N/A**
What size is the water container? ____ **A pool approx 2′ square
and 9″ deep** (60 × 60 × 23 cm)

SOCIAL GROUPING

What other individuals of the same or different
species share the accommodation? _____ **More iguanas**
How many are there of each and of what sex? __ **2 × females in
total**
Do they tend to mix with or ignore each
other? _____ **Sometimes on their own,
at other times together. No sign of aggression etc.**
Is there at least one hide per individual? _____ **Yes**

COOLING DOWN

Please describe this process as fully as possible giving details on
when, for how long, heating, lighting, feeding, disturbances etc.
_____ **N/A**

ANY OTHER COMMENTS

**Both iguanas have a bath in my bath for as long as they
want (usually about 20 mins) twice a week.**

**They also come out of the vivarium regularly and spend time
with the family in both house and garden.**

**They have an 'aviary' type run in the garden which they can
go into on sunny days when we are in the garden.**

HISTORY

SNAKES & LIZARDS – BEARDED DRAGON

ANIMAL'S DETAILS

Name _____**Darwin**

Species (and subspecies if known) _____ **Inland Bearded Dragon/Pogona vitticeps**

Sex _____ **Male**

Where did you get it from? _____ **Reptile Shop**

Approximate age _____**2 yrs** (av. life span 15 – 20 years)

How long have you had it? _____ **1½ years**

When and with what was it last wormed? _____ **6 months ago with Panacur**

HOUSING

VIVARIUM

What is the vivarium made of?_____ **Contiplas wood & glass**

What are its measurements? _____ **8′L × 18″H × 2′D (244 × 46 × 61 cm)**

How is ventilation provided? _____ **Ventilation grills 4″ × 6″ (10 × 15 cm), one in the front at the top the other at the opposite side at the bottom**

LIGHTING

Is there any UV provision? (State type of tube used and how frequently it is changed) _____ **Arcadia D3 lamp changed every 6 months**

How high above the substrate is the UV positioned? _____ **6″ (15 cm) above basking spot**

Is there a spotlight/basking light? (State type
& wattage) _____ **There are two spot lights of**
150 W. Reduced to 60 W during cooling down
Does the spotlight/basking light have a guard around it? ___ **Yes**
How long are each of the lights on for each day:
   Summer _____ **14 hours**
   Winter _____ **10 hours**

HEATING

What type of heater is used? _____ **Tubular greenhouse heater**
Does it have a guard around it? _____ **Yes**
Is it connected to a thermostat? _____ **Yes**
State the background temperatures: Summer   Winter
   Day _____ **27–33°C**   **20–25°C**
   Night _____ **22–24°C**   **18–20°C**
Do you use min./max. thermometers? _____ **Yes**
What is the temperature under the spotlight/basking light? __ **38°C**
Is all the heating and lighting equipment at the
same end of the vivarium? _____ **Yes**
What is the temperature difference between
the hot end and the cool end? _____ **approx. 5°C**

HUMIDITY

What is the humidity? _____ **Varies between 30 and 40%**
Is there a humidity gauge? _____ **Yes**
How is it provided? _____ **Light spraying daily**

DÉCOR

What substrate is used? ___ **calci-sand & potting compost mix**
How deep is the substrate? _____ **Approx. 1″ (2.5 cm)**
How frequently is the vivarium cleaned out? _____ **Approx. every**
2 weeks
What cleaning solution is used? _____ **Milton sterilising fluid**

Describe the hide box/es _____ **Shredded paper, Habba Hut (proprietary bark-like hide), wood**

Is there a covered, damp moss/peat container? _____ **Yes**

What other items of décor are there?

(rocks, branches, drain pipes, plants –

plastic or real etc,) _____ **Slate ramps to heater guard, large branches**

FEEDING

List **all** food items fed & how often each is given (if fruit & vegetables list each type) _____ **See attached diet sheet. Fruit/veg./leafy greens. A selection from the following: Rocket, basil, coriander, dandelion leaves & flowers, clover leaves & flowers, kiwi, peaches, melon, apricot, pear, blackberries, grapes, broccoli, cauliflower, peas, runner beans & leaves, chard, mange tout, water cress, sweetcorn.**

How often is the animal fed? _____ **As over**

What supplements are provided and how often? _____ **Nutrobal**

If feeding with insects, how do you ensure the supplement is delivered? _____ **Crickets are fed directly to him using plastic tweezers**

What are the insects fed on? _____ **Cricket diet plus**

What size is the water container? _____ **Bowl about 3″ (7.5 cm) diameter**

SOCIAL GROUPING

What other individuals of the same or different species share the accommodation? _____ **One other B. dragon**

How many are there of each and of what sex? _____ **Female**

Do they tend to mix with or ignore each other? _ **They mix well**

Is there at least one hide per individual? _____ **Yes**

Table 2.1 Weekly diet sheet. Species. Bearded Dragon 'Darwin'

DAY	FOOD	QUANTITY	SUPPLEMENT
MONDAY	Crickets Fruit/veg./leafy greens	4 Small handful shared between both dragons	Yes No
TUESDAY	Fruit/veg./leafy greens	Large handful between both	No
WEDNESDAY	B. Dragon pellets Fruit/veg./leafy greens	Approx. 15/20 Small handful between both	Yes No
THURSDAY	Crickets Fruit/veg./leafy greens	4 Small handful between both	Yes No
FRIDAY	Fruit/veg./leafy greens	Large handful between both	No
SATURDAY	Waxworms OR small snails Fruit/veg./leafy greens	4 4 Small handful between both	No No Yes
SUNDAY	Crickets Fruit/veg./leafy greens	4 Small handful between both	Yes No

COOLING DOWN

At the beginning of December I start to reduce the background temperatures until they reach 20–25°C during the day and 18–20°C at night. The spotlight/basking light is also reduced in wattage until it reaches 30°C underneath. The lighting cycle is reduced to 10 hours of daylight. This is maintained for about 6 weeks then I start to reverse the process. The whole procedure takes about 10 weeks

_____

_____

_____

_____

ANY OTHER COMMENTS

_____

_____

_____

_____

_____

_____

_____

HISTORY

TORTOISES – SPUR-THIGHED

[IF THE TORTOISE IS KEPT IN A VIVARIUM INSIDE THE HOUSE USE THE HISTORY FORM FOR SNAKES & LIZARDS]

ANIMAL'S DETAILS

Name _____ **Dudley**

Species _____ **Spur-thighed Tortoise/Testudo gracea**

Sex _____ **Male**

Where did you get it from? _____ **Friend**

Approximate age _____ **Unknown but at least 15 yrs**

(av. life span 50–100yrs)

How long have you had it? _____ **2 yrs**

When and with what was it last wormed? _____ **Wormed in September & March each year with Panacur**

HOUSING

HOUSE

Describe the housing and run. Include approximate size, construction materials and a diagram if applicable. (If there is more than one accommodation type provided, fill in a separate form for each)

House is constructed of half round logs on the outside and contiplas board on the inside. There is a 3″ (7.5 cm) gap between the two which is filled with fibreglass insulation. The whole of the roof is hinged and lifts up to allow access for cleaning etc. This is covered with roofing felt. The house is about 4′ × 4′ and 3′ high (1.2 × 1.2 × 1.0 m). There is a 'pop hole' at the front, about 9″ (23 cm) square, that has a solid door

which can be opened or closed. **Inside the door are strips of a tough plastic material covering the aperture so that the heat is retained inside but the tortoise can push through to gain access via a small ramp into the run. The run is also constructed of half round logs and is about 4′ wide 10′ long and 1½′ high** (1.2 × 3.0 × 0.5 m). **There is a small, shallow concrete pond sunk into the corner. The run has rocks and small hillocks and contains long grass to hide in. [See Fig. 2.1]**

During inclement weather is the tortoise shut in its house or does it still have access to the outside? ____ **Has access to the outside all of the summer but not during the winter**

LIGHTING

Is there any UV provision? (State type used & how frequently it is changed) _____ **Reptiglo 5.0, changed once a year as access to sun in summer**

How high above 'tortoise level' is it placed? _____ **9″ (23 cm)**

Is there a spotlight/basking light?
(State type & wattage) _____ **Repti-basking spot, 100 w.**

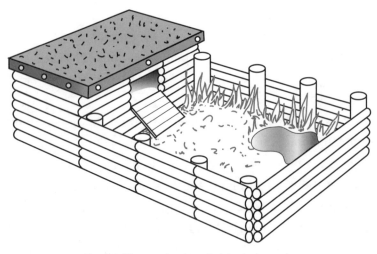

Fig. 2.1 Diagram showing a tortoise house and run

For how long are the lights on each day? _____ **When not hibernating, 14 hrs**

HEATING

What type of heater is used? _____ **Tubular greenhouse heater**

Does it have a guard around it? _____ **Yes**

Is it connected to a thermostat? _____ **Yes**

What is the background temperature? Day **30°C** Night ____ **25°C**

What is the temperature variation between the hot and cold

sections? _____ **Within the house 2–3°C, outside can be quite a lot**

What is the temperature under the

spotlight/basking light? _____ **35°C**

What type of thermometer is used? _____ **Min./max.**

DÉCOR

What substrate is used? ____ **Finely chopped straw, shredded paper and good quality hay**

How frequently is it cleaned out? _____ **As necessary; usually every 2 months**

What cleaning solution is used? _____ **Hibiscrub**

Describe the hide box/es ____ **Hay & paper in the house. Long grass & rock cave outside**

If there a special area for egg laying,

describe it. _____ **An area of the run is kept as bare earth.**

FEEDING

List **all** types of food items given including quantity

and frequency *or* complete a diet sheet _____ **See diet sheet.**

Fruit & veg. mix is chopped into small pieces and a selection from: red apple, pear, melon, peach,

**banana, cabbage, pak choi, curly kale,
spinach, broccoli, cauliflower, cooked carrot,
swede, courgette, baby sweetcorn, asparagus,
runner beans & leaves, peas, cucumber,
cress, mushroom, cherry tomato**

State approximately how much is given on
a daily basis _____ **As below.**

What supplements are given and
how often? _____ **Nutrobal, see diet sheet**

Table 2.2 Weekly diet sheet. Species. Spur-thighed Tortoise 'Dudley'			
DAY	FOOD/S	AMOUNT	SUPPLEMENT State type
MONDAY	Dandelion flowers & leaves, clover etc. for pref., else, a mix of herbs (basil, coriander, rocket, etc.)	A handful per tortoise	Nutrobal
TUESDAY	Fruit & vegetable mix	As above	
WEDNESDAY	Soaked herbivore pellets	A dessert spoon (when dry) per tortoise	Nutrobal
THURSDAY	Fruit & vegetable mix	A handful per tortoise	
FRIDAY	As for Monday	As above	Nutrobal
SATURDAY	Fruit & vegetable mix	As above	
SUNDAY	As for Wednesday	A dessert spoon (when dry) per tortoise	Nutrobal

SOCIAL GROUPING

What other individuals of the same or different species share the
accommodation? (State how many there are of each and of
what sex) _____ **2 more spur-thighs. In total
2 × males & 1 × female**

Describe how they interact with each other _____ **Dudley**
spends some of his time trying to mate the other two.
Sometimes they all sleep together, other times they find
separate places to be.

HIBERNATION

If you provide a gradual cooling down prior to hibernation please
describe the process.

The temperature in the house is decreased by about 2–3°C
each week initially, then by 5°C until it is turned off completely.
At the same time, the lighting time is reduced by about 15
mins a week at each end of the day. The spotlight is reduced
to a 60 w then 40 w bulb, then turned off completely during
the day and replaced with a red light at night that will come
on if the temp. falls to 1°C. The tortoises are still allowed
access into the run initially as the only food available is grass,
which they will not eat. Once the temp. reaches 20°C they are
shut inside. The bedding is changed to newspaper and plenty
of shredded paper that completely fills the house. When the
heating is turned off the temperature in the house does not
rise above 10°C in the winter. If it goes below 1°C the red light
will come on automatically to provide just enough heat to
keep the temp. above freezing. After about 3 months the
heating & lighting are gradually increased until they wake up.
Then returned to normal settings. They stay inside the house
until the weather warms up.

For how long is food withheld prior to
entering hibernation? _____ **5/6 weeks**
Do you worm the tortoise prior to hibernation? _____ **Yes**
If you weigh the tortoise prior to hibernation
what criteria do you use for deciding whether
to hibernate or not? _____ **Jackson's Ratio**

Describe the hibernation accommodation
and siting in detail _____ **See above**

How often do you check the tortoise
during hibernation? _____ **Visual check every week,**
weigh them every month or so.

At the end of hibernation do you
wake the tortoise yourself or
allow it to wake up itself? _____ **Wake them up myself**

If it wakes up by itself how do you know
when it has done so? _____ **Make daily checks as**
the temperature warms up

Please describe what you do immediately
the tortoise has woken up and for the
following few days

Once they are fully awake they are brought into the house and
bathed then put back into their house with full heating &
lighting. A small amount of food is offered for the first couple
of days then normal quantities after that.

ANY OTHER COMMENTS

_____

_____

_____

_____

_____

_____

_____

_____

HISTORY

TERRAPINS – RED-EARED

ANIMAL'S DETAILS

Name _____ **Snoopy**

Species (and subspecies if known)_____**Red-eared Terrapin/**
Trachemys scripta elegans

Sex _____ **Female**

Where did you get it from? _____ **Friend**

Approximate age _____ **12 – 15 years** (av. life span 30–40 yrs)

How long have you had it? _____ **8 years**

When and with what was it last wormed? _____ **2 months ago**
with panacur 10%

HOUSING

Please fill in the relevant section (inside/outside). If the terrapin is
housed both outside and inside at different times of the year fill
in both sections and specify when each is applicable.

OUTSIDE

Describe the accommodation, including measurements and
depth of the pond and the whole enclosure.

**The pen is about 10′ × 10′ (3 m × 3 m). There is a concrete pond
in the middle which is 7′ × 6′ and 2′ (2.1 × 1.8 × 0.6 m) deep.
One end is gently sloping and roughened to allow easy
access into and out of the pond. There is a gentle waterfall
which trickles a constant supply of fresh water during the
day; the overflow is drained away by an overflow pipe. The
area surrounding the pond is long grass and a few large**

rocks. The wire fence is 5′ (152 cm) **high and dug 8″** (20 cm) **into the ground.**

_____

_____

_____

Does the terrapin overwinter in the pond? _____ **No**

If so, how deep is the mud at the bottom? _____ **N/A**

INSIDE

Describe the set-up including measurements of the overall accommodation and the water area.

A water tank measuring 4′ × 4′ × 3½′ (122 × 122 × 106 cm) **deep. The water is 2½′** (76 cm) **deep. At one end there is a ledge which extends all the way across and is 1½′** (46 cm) **wide and lined with astro-turf. There is a ramp that leads from the water to the ledge.**

Describe the access from the water to the land area __ **See above**

What is the substrate on the land area? _____ **Astro-turf**

LIGHTING

Is there any UV provision? (State type of

tube used and how frequently it is changed) _____ **Reptisun 5.0**

changed every winter

How high above the substrate/water is

the UV positioned? _____ **Suspended 1′** (30 cm)

above the land area

Is there a spotlight/basking light?

(State type & wattage) _____ **100w reflector**

For how long are the lights on each day? _____ **12 hours**

What is the temperature of the water? _____ **20–22°C**

How is this maintained? (state type of

heater if used) _____ **No heater is used as the**

room is heated both day and night

What type of thermometer is used to monitor the water
temperature? _____ **Submersible aquarium thermometer**
Does the water heater have a guard around it? _____ **N/A**
Is it connected to a thermostat? _____ **N/A**
What is the background temperature
in the accommodation? _____ **The tank is not enclosed,
therefore it is the same as the room (approx. 25°C)**
How is this maintained? (state type of heater if used)
_____ **N/A**
Does the background heater have a guard around it? _____ **N/A**
Is it connected to a thermostat? _____ **N/A**
Do you use a min./max. thermometer in
the accommodation _____ **Yes**
What is the temperature under the
spotlight/basking light? _____ **32°C**

WATER

This applies to both inside and outside accommodation
What type of (and capacity) filter is used? ___ **External canister
(Green genie 6000) moves 660 gallons per hour**
How often is the water changed – partially? __ **The water is not
changed partially but it is skimmed for debris daily**
totally? _____ **Once a week inside, every 2 weeks outside**
Describe the process for changing
the water _____ **Inside the water is siphoned
out. Outside it is drained through a 'plug hole'**
Is the pond natural and self-sustaining? _____ **No**

FEEDING

How often is the terrapin fed? _____ **Every other day
they get a proper feed but on
the other days they get a small**

amount of floating sticks to provide
them with environmental enrichment
List **all** food items given, including quantity
and frequency, *or* complete a diet sheet _____ **See diet sheets**
for an example of feeding regime

Table 2.3 Weekly diet sheet – Week 1. Species: Red-eared Terrapin, 'Snoopy'.			
DAY	*FOOD/S*	*AMOUNT*	*SUPPLEMENT* *State type*
MONDAY	Fish	2 small (2"/5 cm long)	Ark-vits
TUESDAY	Floating sticks	5 each[a]	
WEDNESDAY	Crickets	4	
THURSDAY	Floating sticks	5 each[a]	
FRIDAY	Pinkies	1	Ark-vits
SATURDAY	Cabbage/lettuce leaf	1 leaf	
SUNDAY	Worms/snails	3	

[a] Terrapin shares accommodation with another female. Floating sticks not fed
to them individually

Table 2.4 Weekly diet sheet – Week 2. Species: Red-eared Terrapin 'Snoopy'			
DAY	*FOOD/S*	*AMOUNT*	*SUPPLEMENT* *State type*
MONDAY	Floating sticks	5 each[a]	
TUESDAY	Prawns	2	Ark-vits
WEDNESDAY	Cabbage leaf		
THURSDAY	Crickets	4	
FRIDAY	Floating sticks	5 each[a]	
SATURDAY	Banana	2 slices (approx. 1 cm wide)	Ark-vits
SUNDAY	Floating sticks	5 each[a]	

[a] Terrapin shares accommodation with another female. Floating sticks not fed
to them individually

What supplements are provided and how often? _____ **Ark vits;**

see sheet

How do you ensure the supplement is delivered? ___ **See below**

What are the insects fed on? _____ **Fruit & vegetables**

Describe the method of feeding (e.g. throw food

into the water, hand-fed etc.) _____ **All food except the floating**

sticks is given to them using tweezers

SOCIAL GROUPING

How many other terrapins share the

accommodation? – male _____ **None**

female _____ **One**

Are they all the same species? _____ **Yes**

ANY OTHER COMMENTS

The terrapins spend the winter in the inside accommodation. In late spring as the weather warms up they are put outside on fine days and brought in at night. In the summer, when the weather has warmed up sufficiently, they are left outside day and night. When the weather starts to turn cold in the late summer/early autumn they are brought in for the winter.

HISTORY

AMPHIBIANS – FIRE-BELLIED TOAD

ANIMAL'S DETAILS

Name _____ **Toady**

Species (and subspecies if known) _____ **Oriental fire bellied toad/Bombina orientalis**

Sex _____ **Male**

Where did you get it from? _____ **Pet shop**

Approximate age _____ **2 yrs** (av. life span 12–15 yrs)

How long have you had it? _____ **1 yr**

HOUSING

VIVARIUM

What is the vivarium made of? **Glass, all sides except the front and top covered with polystyrene sheets**

What are its measurements? _____ **2′6″ l × 2′w × 1′6″ h** (76 × 61 × 46 cm)

How is ventilation provided? _____ **Half the lid is wire mesh**

Where is the vivarium sited? _____ **Corner of dining room away from window and heater**.

LIGHTING

What type of lighting is provided? _____ **Full spectrum-Reptisun 2.0, spotlight/basking light**

What wattage is it? _____ **Spotlight/basking light – 40W**

How high above the highest surface is it? _____ **9 inches** (23 cm)

Does it have a guard around it? _____ **Yes**

For how long are the lights on each day? _____ **12 hours**

HEATING

What is the temperature of the water? _____ **Approx. 24–25°C**

How is this maintained? (state type of
heater is used) _____ **Aquarium heater**

What type of thermometer is used to monitor the water
temperature? _____ **Floating aquarium
thermometer**

Does the water heater have a guard around it? _____ **Yes**

Is it connected to a thermostat? ____ **Has a built-in thermostat**

What is the background temperature in the accommodation?

Day _____ **26–28°C**

Night _____ **22–24°C**

How is this maintained? (state type
of heater if used) _____ **Heat pads along one end
and half of the back
wall (land area)**

Does the background heater have
a guard around it? _____ **On outside of glass**

Is it connected to a thermostat? _____ **Yes**

Do you use a min./max. thermometer in
the accommodation? _____ **Yes**

What is the temperature under the spotlight/basking light? ___ **32°C**

HUMIDITY

What is the humidity? _____ **Between 50 and 60%**

Is there a humidity gauge? _____ **Yes**

DÉCOR – LAND

What proportion of the vivarium is land area? _____ **One end
of the tank, approx. a third**

What substrate is used? _____ **Sterilised moss**

How deep is the substrate? _____ **About ½″ (1 cm)**

How is the humidity/dampness maintained? ____ **Daily spraying**

Describe the land area (include items of furniture and method of access from the water) _____ **2′ front to back × 9″ long. Access into water is by a sloping slate. There is a clay drainpipe cut in half lengthways, a piece of tree root, a piece of cork bark and plants**

Are there any plants? (specify whether real or plastic) _____ **Both**

If real, what species are they? _____ **Bromeliads**

Have they been re-potted into soil? _____ **Yes**

Is a spotlight/basking light provided? (give details) ____ **Yes 40w spotlight**

How frequently is the vivarium cleaned out? _____ **The moss is washed every week and changed monthly**

What cleaning solution is used? _____ **Hot, dechlorinated water**

DÉCOR – WATER

How large is the water area? _____ **2′ front to back × 1′9″ long** (61 × 53 cm)

How deep is the water? _____ **approx. 4″** (10 cm)

What substrate is used? _____ **Large gravel**

What other items of décor are there? (e.g. logs, rocks, drainpipes etc.) _____ **Rocks (protruding above the surface), 'mopani' root** (specialist aquarium wood that sinks to the bottom), **plastic plants**

Is there a water filter? [If yes state type (undergravel, internal, external) and capacity] ___ **Internal – Fluval 1, 45 litre capacity**

How is the water dechlorinated? _____ **Zoo Med Reptisafe**

How often is the water changed? **Partial weekly, total monthly**

FEEDING

List **all** food items fed, how much and how often each is given _____ **2 × crickets – 2/3 times weekly; 2 × waxworms – weekly; 1 × garden worm**

chopped up – occasionally, daphnia – occasionally
(lots released into the water), approx
1 × teasp. of blood worm – occasionally

How often is the animal fed? _____ **Every other day**

What supplements are provided and how often? _____ **Reptavite**

If feeding with insects, how do you ensure the supplement is
delivered? _____ **Mostly hand-fed**

What are the insects fed on? _____ **Fish flakes & apple**

SOCIAL GROUPING

Does it live alone or with other individuals? (state species &
numbers) _____ **Six other fire-bellies**

What is the ratio of sexes, if known? _____ **3 × female, 4 × male**

HANDLING

How frequently is it handled? _____ **Seldom**

Describe how this is done _____ **Very carefully! With wet,**
disposable gloves

COOLING DOWN

Please describe fully the process of cooling down, length of
cooling and warming back up.

Over a couple of weeks the temperature is lowered to about
15/16°C, kept there for about a month and then brought back
up to normal. This species does not undergo a proper
hibernation (as do other Bombina species) just a lowering of the
overall temperatures.

ANY OTHER COMMENTS

_____

_____

_____

AUTHOR'S NOTE – BOMBINA SPECIES

There are three Bombina species that are commonly kept, each requiring slightly different conditions, mostly relating to temperature. It is important therefore to correctly establish the species in question.

This is not the place to go into detail about specific species identification and care. (There are good books and internet articles covering this information.) However, below is a brief description of each, which illustrates how easy it is to confuse the species.

1   Bombina orientalis (Oriental fire-bellied toad)
    Have red and black bellies. However, captive bred ones may have **yellow** and black bellies. This can be rectified by feeding them beta carotene (often used by canary breeders to keep their colour).

2   Bombina variegata (Yellow-bellied toad)
    As the name implies, these have yellow bellies.

3   Bombina bombina (European fire-bellied toad)
    This species also has a red and black ventral area and again, as with B. orientalis, this may become orange or yellow in captivity.

HISTORY

AMPHIBIANS – HORNED FROG

ANIMAL'S DETAILS

Name _____ **Jabba the Hut**

Species (and subspecies if known) _____ **Ornate horned frog/**
Ceratophrys ornata

Sex _____ **Male**

Where did you get it from? _____ **Friend**

Approximate age _____ **4 yrs** (av. life span 7–10 yrs)

How long have you had it? _____ **2½ yrs**

HOUSING

VIVARIUM

What is the vivarium made of? _____ **Glass**

What are its measurements? __ **2′l × 1′w × 1′h** (61 × 30 × 30 cm)

How is ventilation provided? _____ **Lid is half mesh**

Where is the vivarium sited? _____ **Bedroom**

LIGHTING

What type of lighting is provided? ___ **Arcadia natural sun light**

What wattage is it? _____ **18W**

How high above the highest surface is it? __ **Approx. 7″** (18 cm)

Does it have a guard around it? _____ **Not necessary**

For how long are the lights on each day? _____ **12 hours**

HEATING

What is the temperature of the water? _____ **Warm**

How is this maintained? (state type of

heater if used) _____ **Air temp. in vivarium**

What type of thermometer is used to
monitor the water temperature? ___ **None, it's only a small dish**

Does the water heater have a guard around it? _____ **N/A**

Is it connected to a thermostat? _____ **N/A**

What is the background temperature in the accommodation?

  Day _____ **28°C**

  Night _____ **24°C**

How is this maintained? (state type of heater if used) _ **Heat mats
under half the floor area and along half of the back wall**

Does the background heater have a guard
around it? _____ **On outside of vivarium**

Is it connected to a thermostat? _____ **Yes**

Do you use a min./max. thermometer in
the accommodation? _____ **Yes**

What is the temperature under the spotlight? _____ **N/A**

HUMIDITY

What is the humidity? _____ **80%**

Is there a humidity gauge? _____ **Yes**

DÉCOR – LAND

What proportion of the vivarium is land area? _____ **Most of it**

What substrate is used? _____ **Terrarium moss & clean,
sterilised top soil**

How deep is the substrate? _____ **Approx. 2–3 inches** (6 cm)

How is the humidity/dampness maintained? _____ **Spraying
twice a day**

Describe the land area (include items of furniture & method of
access from the water) _____ **Piece of cork bark just large
enough for him to get under, tree root, rocks
forming a cave, water dish sunk into substrate**

Are there any plants? (specify whether real or plastic) __ **Plastic**

If real, what species are they? _____ **N/A**

Have they been re-potted into soil? _____ **N/A**

Is a spotlight/basking light provided? (give details) _____ **No**

How frequently is the vivarium cleaned out? _____ **Partially**
every 2/3 days, totally every month
(depending on how active he has been and
how much of the vivarium has been used)

What cleaning solution is used? _____ **Hot, dechlorinated water**

DÉCOR – WATER

How large is the water area? _____ **Shallow dish approx.**
8 inches (20 cm) **in diameter**

How deep is the water? _____ **about 1½ inches** (4 cm)

What substrate is used? _____ **None**

What other items of décor are there? (e.g. logs, rocks,
drainpipes, etc.) _____ **plastic plant for shelter/hide**

Is there a water filter? [if yes, state type(undergravel, internal,
external) and capacity] _____ **No**

How is the water dechlorinated? _____ **Stands for three days**

How often is the water changed? _____ **Daily**

FEEDING

List **all** food items fed, how
much and how often each is given _____ **3 × Crickets – twice a**
week; 1 × pinky (baby mouse) – every
three weeks; 1 × small fish – every three weeks;
2 × waxworms – every three weeks

How often is the animal fed? _____ **3 × a week**

What supplements are provided
and how often? _____ **Reptavite on crickets**

If feeding with insects, how do you ensure the supplement is
delivered? _____ **All food is fed using tweezers**

What are the insects fed on? _____ **Bug Grub**

SOCIAL GROUPING

Does it live alone or with other individuals? (state species &
numbers) _____ **On his own**
What is the ratio of sexes, if known? _____ **N/A**

HANDLING

How frequently is it handled? __ **Only to move it when cleaning**
Describe how this is done _____ **Wash hands in hot**
water, then rinse with de-chlorinated water.
Whilst hands are still wet frog is scooped up in
both hands and transferred to separate container

COOLING DOWN

Please describe fully the process of cooling down,
length of cooling and warming back up. _____ **N/A**

ANY OTHER COMMENTS

_____
_____
_____
_____
_____
_____
_____
_____
_____
_____
_____
_____
_____
_____
_____

AUTHOR'S NOTE – HORNED FROGS

Some points to bear in mind about this species:

1   They are very poor swimmers, therefore the water should be just deep enough to cover them about half way.
2   Light bulbs tend to dry them out quickly, so if they are used it should be with care.
3   They require high humidity.
4   They should be kept singly as they have a tendency to eat each other!

HISTORY

AMPHIBIANS – WHITE'S TREE FROG

ANIMAL'S DETAILS

Name _____ **Humpty**

Species (and subspecies if known) _____ **White's tree frog/**

Litoria caerulea

Sex _____ **Female**

Where did you get it from? _____ **Breeder**

Approximate age _____ **5 yrs** (av. life span 10–15 yrs)

How long have you had it? _____ **4½ yrs**

HOUSING

VIVARIUM

What is the vivarium made of? _____ **Fibre glass**

What are its measurements? ___ **2′l × 2′d × 3′h** (61 × 61 × 92 cm)

How is ventilation provided? ___ **Half of lid is mesh, also mesh**

ventilation panel 2″ × 4″ (5 × 10 cm)

on one side at the bottom

Where is the vivarium sited? _____ **Corner of living room**

(away from windows, radiators & television)

LIGHTING

What type of lighting is provided? ____ **Incandescent light bulb,**

plus full spectrum light tube

What wattage is it?_____ **Light bulb – 60 W, tube**

– Arcadia tube 18 W

How high above the highest surface is it? ____ **Both lights are**

outside vivarium hanging over mesh part of lid

Does it have a guard around it? _____ **N/A**

How long are the lights on each day? ___ **Light bulb – 12 hours, tube – 2 hours (for the plants)**

HEATING

What is the temperature of the water? _____ **Room temperature**

How is this maintained? (state type of heater if used) _____ **ambient temperature of the vivarium**

What type of thermometer is used to monitor the water temperature? _____ **None**

Does the water heater have a guard around it? _____ **N/A**

Is it connected to a thermostat?_____ **N/A**

What is the background temperature in the accommodation?

  Day _____ **25°C**

  Night _____ **20°C**

How is this maintained? (State type of heater if used) _____ **Heat mats covering the entire back wall and half of one side-wall (full height)**

Does the background heater have a guard around it? _____ **Mats on outside of vivarium**

Is it connected to a thermostat? _____ **Yes**

Do you use a min./max. thermometer in the accommodation? _____ **Yes**

What is the temperature under the spotlight? _____ **30°C**

HUMIDITY

What is the humidity? _____ **50–60%**

Is there a humidity gauge? _____ **Yes**

DÉCOR – LAND

What proportion of the vivarium is land area? _____ **Most of it**

What substrate is used? _____ **Clean top soil & terrarium moss**

How deep is the substrate? _____ **approx. ½″ − 1″** (1–2 cm)

How is humidity/dampness maintained? _ **Spraying twice daily**

Describe the land area. (Include items of
furniture & method of access from the water) _____ **Tall bits
of cork bark placed against walls to
provide dark hiding places, sloping
tree branches, plants. Water is a
shallow bowl**

Are there any plants? (Specify whether real or plastic) ____ **Both**

If real, what species are they? _____ **Mother-in-law's tongue**

Have they been re-potted into soil? _____ **Yes**

Is a spotlight/basking light provided?
(Give details) _____ **Incandescent
bulb as described earlier**

How frequently is the vivarium
cleaned out? _____ **Sides wiped daily, full clean
out every 2–3 weeks**

What cleaning solution is used? ____ **Hot, dechlorinated water**

DÉCOR – WATER

How large is the water area? _____ **8″ (20 cm) round shallow
dish, with gently sloping sides**

How deep is the water? _____ **deep enough to come
about ¾ of the way up the frog
when sitting in it**

What substrate is used? _____ **None**

What other items of décor are there?
(logs, rocks, drainpipes etc.) _____ **None**

Is there a water filter? (if yes state type
(undergravel, internal, external) and capacity) _____ **N/A**

How is the water dechlorinated? _____ **Left to stand for
at least three days**

How often is the water changed? _____ **Daily**

FEEDING

List **all** food items fed, how much
and how often each is given _____ **2 or 3 crickets hand-fed
at two out of every three feeds and
about 12 released into the vivarium;
1 or 2 waxworms every third feed. Amounts
vary depending on appetite and weight**
How often is the animal fed? _____ **Usually three times a week**
What supplements are provided and how often? _____ **Nutrobal**
If feeding with insects, how do you
ensure the supplement is delivered? _____ **They are hand-fed**
What are the insects fed on? _____ **Fruit & vegetables**

SOCIAL GROUPING

Does it live alone or with other individuals?
(State species & numbers) _____ **Six White's altogether**
What is the ratio of sexes, if known? _____ **Unsure, but
think three of each**

HANDLING

How frequently is it handled? _____ **Once or twice a week
and when cleaning**
Describe how this is done _____ **Hands washed in hot
water then rinsed in dechlorinated
water and kept wet while handling.
Hands washed with antibacterial
soap afterwards**

COOLING DOWN

Please describe fully the process of cooling down, length of
cooling and warming back up _____ **N/A**

ANY OTHER COMMENTS

_____

_____

_____

_____

_____

_____

_____

_____

AUTHOR'S NOTE – WHITE'S TREE FROGS

1   If all-glass vivariums are used it can create a problem with the frogs trying to 'get through' the glass at the bottom and damaging the skin around the nose and mouth. As already mentioned in the explanation of questions, covering three of the sides with an opaque material should be done anyway to give a sense of security. If the uncovered front section still is a problem, placing a strip of dark paper about 4/5 inches (12 cm) deep along the front at the bottom should stop the behaviour.

2   As this species is nocturnal they tend to hide away from bright light. Having said this, they do seem to enjoy basking on occasions, therefore a spotlight/basking lamp is a good idea, particularly if a piece of cork or a branch can be arranged so that there is a temperature gradient. (Fig. 2.2)

3   These frogs are not strong swimmers so it is not a good idea to give them a large or deep water area.

4   White's seem to tolerate handling far better than most amphibians, providing it is done carefully and not too frequently.

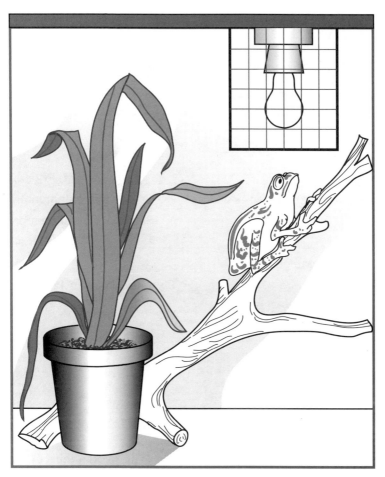

Fig. 2.2 Diagram showing branch for temperature gradient

HISTORY

AMPHIBIANS – FIRE SALAMANDER

ANIMAL'S DETAILS

Name _____ **Phoenix**

Species (and subspecies if known) _____ **Fire salamander/ Salamandra salamandra**

Sex _____ **Female**

Where did you get it from? _____ **Pet shop**

Approximate age _____ **8 yrs (**av. life span 12–20 yrs)

How long have you had it? _____ **7 yrs**

HOUSING

VIVARIUM

What is the vivarium made of? _____ **Glass**

What are the measurements of the vivarium? ___ **3′l × 2′w × 1½h** (91 × 61 × 46 cm)

How is ventilation provided?_____ **The middle third of the lid is solid but the two ends are mesh**

Where is the vivarium sited? _____ **Living room**

LIGHTING

What type of lighting is provided? _____ **Arcadia natural sunlight lamp.**

What wattage is it? _____ **18W**

How high above the highest surface is it? _____ **1′ (30 cm)**

Does it have a guard around it? _____ **No, not necessary**

For how long are the lights on each day? _____ **11 hours**

HEATING

What is the temperature of the water? _____ **Not heated, same as vivarium temp.**

How is this maintained? (state type of heater if used) _____ **N/A**

What type of thermometer is used to monitor the water temperature _____ **N/A**

Does the water heater have a guard around it? _____ **N/A**

Is it connected to a thermostat? _____ **N/A**

What is the background temperature in the accommodation?

Day _____ **17–20°C**

Night _____ **12–15°C**

How is this maintained? (State type of heater if used) _____ **Heat mats along one end and half of back wall**

Does the background heater have a guard around it? _____ **On outside of tank**

Is it connected to a thermostat? _____ **Yes, Habistat mat stat**

Do you use a min./max. thermometer in the accommodation? _____ **Yes**

What is the temperature under the spotlight? ___ **There isn't one**

HUMIDITY

What is the humidity? _____ **50–60%**

Is there a humidity gauge? _____ **Yes**

DÉCOR – LAND

What proportion of the vivarium is land area? _____ **Most of it**

What substrate is used? _____ **A layer of sterilised top soil mixed with silver sand covered with a layer of moss**

How deep is the substrate? _____ **Sand & soil layer is about 4″ (10 cm) deep, moss about 1–2″ (3–5 cm) deep**

How is humidity/dampness
maintained? _____ **Regular misting and watering**
Describe the land area. (Include items
of furniture & method of access
from the water) _____ **Contains mopani logs, rocks to hide
under, broken clay pots, cork bark pieces
& plants in pots sunk into the substrate.
Water is very shallow so access is not a problem**
Are there any plants? (Specify whether
real or plastic) _____ **Real**
If real, what species are they? ____ **Philodendron & bromeliads**
Have they been re-potted into soil? _____ **Yes**
Is a spotlight/basking light provided? (Give details) _____ **No**
How frequently is the vivarium
cleaned out? _____ **Total clean out every 2–3 months.**
What cleaning solution is used? _____ **Hot water**

DÉCOR – WATER

How large is the water area? _____ **1′ × 8″ (30 × 10 cm)**
How deep is the water? _____ **1″ (2.5 cm)**
What substrate is used? _____ **Gravel**
What other items of décor are there?
(e.g. logs, rocks, drainpipes, etc.) _____ **Plastic plant**
Is there a water filter? [if yes state type
(undergravel, internal, external) and capacity] _____ **No**
How is the water dechlorinated? _____ **Reptisafe dechlorinator**
How often is the water changed? _____ **Every day**

FEEDING

List **all** food items fed, how much
and how often each is given _____ **3/4 crickets – 2 × a week;
2/3 waxworms – once a fortnight;
2 small slugs – once a fortnight**

How often is the animal fed? _____ **Three times a week**

What supplements are provided and how often? _____ **Nutrobal**

If feeding with insects, how do you ensure

the supplement is delivered _____ **They are hand fed using tweezers.**

What are the insects fed on? _____ **'Bug Grub'**

SOCIAL GROUPING

Does it live alone or with other individuals? (state species & numbers) ___ **Two other fire salamanders of the same species**

What is the ratio of sexes, if known? _____ **1 × male, 2 × females**

HANDLING

How frequently is it handled? _____ **Not very often**

Describe how this is done _____ **Usually when transferring to another container for cleaning etc. They are coaxed into it without actually having to handle them, but if they do have to be handled it is done wearing wet, disposable, polythene gloves**

COOLING DOWN

Please describe fully the process of cooling down, length of cooling and warming back up.

Food is withheld for three weeks before cooling down, then the temperature is gradually reduced over about three weeks to 5°C. The salamanders are then transferred to a small container with damp moss and a water bowl and kept at approx. 5°C for another month, then gradually warmed up and transferred to their permanent enclosure.

ANY OTHER COMMENTS

_____

_____

_____

_____

_____

_____

_____

_____

AUTHOR'S NOTE – FIRE SALAMANDERS

There are many subspecies of fire salamander and their habitats vary, although most can be kept under similar conditions.

1   Salamanders are quite active so require a relatively large vivarium.

2   They are nocturnal and do not require a basking spot, but some form of lighting (even if it is only subdued) is necessary to regulate their day/night cycle.

3   If the temperature is too hot, fire salamanders will display typical behavioural signs of trying to climb the walls and/or circling the tank.

4   Fire salamanders have a line of pores running down either side of the head, back and tail. If the animal is alarmed, these will secrete a milky, alkaloid substance that is not pleasant, especially if it gets into your eyes.

3 SELF-TEST HISTORIES

The following are real life examples. Read through the forms and see what areas you think could be improved, are inappropriate or need further questioning, then check your findings with the author's at the back of each form.

HISTORY

SNAKES & LIZARDS

ANIMAL'S DETAILS

Name _____ **Barty**

Species (and subspecies if known) _____ **Corn snake**

Sex _____ **Male**

Where did you get it from? _____ **Pet shop**

Approximate age _____ **2 years**

How long have you had it? _____ **6 months**

When and with what was it last wormed _____ **Unknown**

HOUSING

VIVARIUM

What is the vivarium made of? _____ **Wood & glass**

What are its measurements? _____ **3′l × 1′d × 1′h**

(92 × 30 × 30 cm)

How is ventilation provided? _____ **Top 3″ (7.5 cm) on**

the back wall is wire mesh

LIGHTING

Is there any UV provision? (State type of tube

used and how frequently it is changed) _____ **No**

How high above the substrate is the

UV positioned? _____ **N/A**

Is there a spotlight/basking light?

(State type & wattage) _____ **100w spotlight**

Does the spotlight/basking light have a guard around it? ___ **Yes**

How long are the lights on each day?

Summer _____ **8.00 am – 8.00 pm**

Winter _____ **as above**

HEATING

What type of heater is used? _____ **Overhead flat trough ceramic**

Does it have a guard around it? _____ **Yes**

Is it connected to a thermostat? _____ **Yes**

State the background temperatures: Summer Winter

   Day _____ **27–30°C** **27–30°C**

   Night _____ **23–25°C** **23–25°C**

Do you use min./max. thermometers? _____ **Yes**

What is the temperature under the
spotlight/basking light? _____ **33°C**

Is all the heating and lighting equipment at
the same end of the vivarium? _____ **Yes**

What is the temperature difference between the
hot end and the cool end? _____ **2–3°C**

HUMIDITY

What is the humidity? _____ **Normal room**

Is there a humidity gauge? _____ **No**

How is it provided? _____ **N/A**

DÉCOR

What substrate is used? _____ **Newspaper**

How deep is the substrate? _____ **4/5 layers**

How frequently is the vivarium cleaned out? _____ **Paper is changed whenever it is dirty**

What cleaning solution is used? _____ **Hibiscrub**

Describe the hide box/es _____ **Cork bark, small cardboard box**

Is there a covered, damp moss/peat container? _____ **No**

What other items of décor are there?
(Rocks, branches, drain pipes, plants–plastic
or real etc) _____ **Branches, stones**

FEEDING

List **all** food items given including quantity and
frequency *or* complete a diet sheet (if fruit and veg.
list each type) _____ **Adult mice, 1 or 2 every week**
How often is the animal fed? _____ **See above**
What supplements are provided and how often? _____ **None**
If feeding with insects, how do you ensure the
supplement is delivered? _____ **N/A**
What are the insects fed on? _____ **N/A**
What size is the water container? ____ **Ceramic dog food bowl**
approx. 9″ (23 cm) **diameter and 4″** (10 cm) **deep**

SOCIAL GROUPING

What other individuals of the same or different
species share the accommodation? _____ **None**
How many are there of
each and of what sex? _____ **N/A**
Do they tend to mix
with or ignore each other? _____ **N/A**
Is there at least one hide per individual? _____ **Yes**

COOLING DOWN

Please describe this process as fully as possible giving
details on when, for how long, heating, lighting, feeding,
disturbances etc. _____ **Do not cool down**

ANY OTHER COMMENTS

_____
_____
_____

_____

_____

_____

_____

_____

COMMENTS

ANIMAL'S DETAILS

- The owner does not know when the snake was last wormed. This implies that it has been at least two years, which is how long it has been with the current owner.

HOUSING

I believe I have already mentioned that I am not an advocate of keeping pet reptiles in small accommodation. Therefore, my comments on this section are commensurate with my own ideas on the subject and not necessarily the opinion of some established reptile keepers.

VIVARIUM

- The vivarium is a little small, particularly in depth and height, to allow sufficient environmental enrichment.
- This method of ventilation is probably OK for this size of vivarium and for this particular species. Because it runs along the entire length of the back wall of fairly small accommodation it is likely to allow sufficient exchange of air, unless, of course, the vivarium is pushed up against a wall.

LIGHTING & HEATING

[*See comments for cooling down.*]

HUMIDITY

- Normal room humidity is usually OK in Britain as it tends to be within the range required by corn snakes, however, if there is no gauge in the vivarium the owner will have no idea if the correct range is being attained.

- It is not necessary to spray with water to maintain the right level of humidity and, provided that there is a peat/moss container, there should not be a problem.

DÉCOR

- There is nothing wrong with newspaper, except that it is not an especially natural substrate and does not really allow for much enrichment.
- Because Barty is a male he does not need an egg-laying chamber but I have found that often both males and females prefer to use a damp area as opposed to a water bowl when sloughing.

SOCIAL GROUPING

- In the wild corn snakes are solitary for the most part but in captivity I feel that company helps to provide stimulation. This species will readily mix with one or more individuals of the same or opposite sex.

COOLING DOWN

- Many corn snakes are kept at the same temperature all year round without apparent detriment. However, North America, which is where this species is found in the wild, has marked seasonal variations and it would seem sensible to recreate this in the captive environment. It may also be that individuals that are not cooled down regularly may have a shortened life span.

HISTORY

SNAKES & LIZARDS

ANIMAL'S DETAILS

Name _____ **Delihla**

Species (and subspecies if known) _____ **Common iguana**

Sex _____ **Female**

Where did you get it from? _____ **Friend**

Approximate age _____ **1½ yrs**

How long have you had it? _____ **1 yr**

When and with what was it

last wormed? _____ **Don't Know**

HOUSING

VIVARIUM

What is the vivarium

made of? _____ **An old wardrobe**

What are its

measurements? _____ **6'high, 2'6 "long, 18" deep**

(1.8 m × 76 cm × 46 cm)

How is ventilation provided? _____ **Small holes drilled in**

both sides

LIGHTING

Is there any UV provision? (State type of tube used and how

frequently it is changed) _____ **She goes for walks**

on a lead outside

most days

How high above the substrate

is the UV positioned? _____ **N/A**

Is there a spotlight/basking light?

(State type & wattage) _____ **100w spotlight**

Does the spotlight/basking light have a guard around it? ___ **Yes**

How long are the lights on each day?

  Summer _____ **12 hours**

  Winter _____ **12 hours**

HEATING

What type of heater is used? _____ **Ceramic heat emitter**

Does it have a guard around it? _____ **Yes**

Is it connected to a thermostat? _____ **Yes**

State the background temperatures: Summer   Winter

  Day _____ **30°C**   **30°C**

  Night _____ **22°C**   **22°C**

Do you use min./max. thermometers? _____ **Yes**

What is the temperature under the

spotlight/basking light? _____ **36°C**

Is all the heating and lighting

equipment at the same end

of the vivarium? _____ **All at the top**

What is the temperature difference

between the hot end and the

cool end? _____ **Between top & bottom – about 7°C**

HUMIDITY

What is the humidity? _____ **Very damp**

Is there a humidity gauge? _____ **No**

How is it provided? _____ **Spraying with water**

at least twice every day

DÉCOR

What substrate is used? _____ **Bark chips**

How deep is the substrate? _____ **About ½″ (1 cm)**

How frequently is the vivarium
cleaned out? _____ **Every 2 weeks**

What cleaning solution is used? _____ **Ark-Klens**

Describe the hide box/es _____ **She has a wooden platform
between two branches
near the top of the cage which
has a bit of curved cork bark on it.**

Is there a covered, damp
moss/peat container? _____ **The floor is covered with
damp bark chips**

What other items of décor are there?
(e.g. rocks, branches, drain pipes, plastic
or real plants, etc. _____ **There are several branches
and some plastic flowers.**

FEEDING

List **all** food items including quantity
and frequency *or* complete the diet
sheet (If fruit & vegetables list each
type) _____ **She has a small bowl of fruit & veg.
every day, e.g. mixed salad leaves
from supermarket and apple.
As well as that she has a few
crickets, or dog food or mealworms**

How often is the animal fed? _____ **Every day**

What supplements are
provided and how often? _____ **Doesn't need any as diet
is varied enough**

If feeding with insects, how do you
ensure the supplement is delivered? _____ **N/A**

What are the insects fed on? _____ **Bran, apple and cabbage**

What size is the water container? _____ **Washing-up bowl**

SOCIAL GROUPING

What other individuals of the same or
different species share the accommodation? _____ **None**

How many are there of each and of what sex? _____ **N/A**

Do they tend to mix with or ignore each other? _____ **N/A**

Is there at least one hide per individual? _____ **Yes**

COOLING DOWN

Please describe fully the process of cooling down,
length of cooling & warming back up. _____ **Doesn't get**
                                                    cooled down

ANY OTHER COMMENTS

_____

_____

_____

_____

_____

_____

_____

_____

COMMENTS

Iguanas should not be kept by a novice keeper. They require spacious accommodation and an understanding of their behaviour and psychology. Rescue centres are full of them because owners take them on without realising what a commitment they are and quickly run into trouble.

ANIMAL'S DETAILS

- Worming is not something that the owners have considered.

HOUSING

VIVARIUM

- Whilst a former wardrobe is not perhaps the ideal form of vivarium it may not be as unsuitable as it sounds, depending on size and the extent to which it has been converted to provide water resistance, adequate ventilation, and so on. However, this particular wardrobe is too small regardless of how well it may have been converted. Rather than messing about with trying to extend it I strongly recommend buying or building a new, more suitable vivarium.

LIGHTING

- Taking her for walks each day is not providing sufficient exposure to UV, even if she is walked for several hours (which is unlikely). Iguanas seem to be more susceptible to metabolic bone disease than other commonly kept species so particular attention must be paid to this aspect. Proper UV lighting must be supplied.
- There is a case for allowing certain species access to an outside run or enclosure (provided that it is set up correctly)

but, personally, I'm not a big fan of taking reptiles for a walk. I think the amount/type of environmental enrichment it provides for the animal is dubious, particularly if these walks take place in public places. Iguanas are intelligent reptiles that require stimulation. Interaction with the owners on a daily basis is definitely a good idea but for the most part this should be restricted to the house and garden.

HEATING

- A ceramic heat emitter is fine in a smaller vivarium, but a single emitter will probably not be able to heat the size of vivarium needed for an iguana. Either several will be needed or an alternative form of heating should be supplied in the new vivarium.
- The night-time temperature is a little low.
- I have already said that this vivarium is unsuitable and should be replaced, however, this gives me an opportunity to discuss a few points relating to temperature gradients that run from top to bottom as opposed to end to end.

1. Such a gradient is going to be unavoidable in a large vivarium but it is not necessarily a problem provided the animal feels comfortable in both the higher and lower areas.
2. Arboreal species like iguanas prefer to be higher up. This may mean that they will not fully utilise all areas of the vivarium.
3. Close observation should be made to assess whether the animal is happy to move about in the lower part. If it is not, the provision of more hides or cover may help them to feel more secure and will encourage them to use, say, the water area more frequently, should they feel so inclined.

HUMIDITY

- 'Very damp' is too subjective. A humidity gauge is needed to accurately judge whether the humidity is appropriate.

DÉCOR

- Because the vivarium is so narrow there is not much room for décor and, consequently, it is a little lacking in items of interest.
- There is a high-level hide which is good, but a selection of hides at various heights would be better.

FEEDING

- Iguanas are herbivorous. In the wild it is quite likely that an insect would be ingested by accident along with a leaf every so often and so, although it is not advocated, it will not harm an iguana to eat the occasional cricket. However, this should not be every day and they definitely must not be given dog food.
- Mixed salad leaves bags usually consist of different types of lettuce. This is also not a good food to be giving too often.
- I would want to know exactly what other fruit and vegetables are given and with what frequency.
- Supplements are a must.
- Bran is not a satisfactory food for the crickets. Apple and cabbage would probably be sufficient to keep them alive but does not really provide sufficient variation to be of much use in gut loading (feeding the cricket with high quality food that will be of nutritional value to the animal that eats the cricket).
- Obviously the owners need some advice about a correct diet.
- If you put together a completely inappropriate diet, no supplementation and a lack of adequate UV provision you have a perfect recipe for advanced metabolic bone disease.

- I would also want to know if the iguana uses the water container as a washing up bowl is probably not large enough for her to fit into easily.

SOCIAL GROUPING

- I prefer not to keep animals on their own as a rule, but keeping two or more iguanas together can be problematic.
- Introducing a new iguana to an existing one is a gamble and depends entirely on individual temperament. There may be no problems at all but, on the other hand, one may be aggressive and dominant. (Females can display dominant behaviour as well as males.) If they have always been housed together this does not mean they will always be compatible either.
- In other words, keeping two iguanas together is preferable and there may be no problems at all, but in some cases you may end up having to build another vivarium.
- Environmental enrichment and interaction with the owners is important to keep these intelligent reptiles occupied, especially if they are kept singly. For example, you should try putting their food in different/several places, letting them out of the vivarium and spending time with them.
- Iguanas (indeed any reptile) should not be allowed out of the vivarium except under supervision, unless you like replacing curtains, ornaments, pot plants, electric cable, other pets, etc.

HISTORY

SNAKES & LIZARDS

ANIMAL'S DETAILS

Name _____ **Poggy**

Species (and subspecies if
known) _____ **Bearded Dragon**

Sex _____ **Male**

Where did you get it from? _____ **Friend**

Approximate age _____ **2 months**

How long have you had it? _____ **2 weeks**

When and with what was it last wormed? _____ **Never**

HOUSING

VIVARIUM

What is the vivarium made of? _____ **Wood & glass**

What are its measurements? **6′l × 2′h × 2′d** (1.8 m × 61 cm × 61 cm)

How is ventilation provided? _____ **Grills at top & bottom
of vivarium**

LIGHTING

Is there any UV provision? (State type of tube used
and how frequently it is changed) _____ **Reptisun 5.0. Not yet
changed it**

How high above the substrate is
the UV positioned? _____ **12″** (30 cm)

Is there a spotlight/basking light?
(State type & wattage) _____ **120W light with
reflector dome**

Does the spotlight/basking light have a guard around it? ____ **No**

For how long are the lights on each day?

Summer _____ **12 hours**

Winter _____ **12 hours**

HEATING

What type of heater is used? _____ **Heat mat**

Does it have a guard around it? _____ **No**

Is it connected to a thermostat? _____ **Yes**

State the background temperatures: Summer Winter

Day _____ **30–34°C** **N/a**

Night _____ **23–25°C** **N/a**

Do you use min./max. thermometers? _____ **Yes**

What is the temperature under
the spotlight/basking light? _____ **39°C**

Is all the heating and lighting equipment at the same
end of the vivarium? _____ **Yes**

What is the temperature difference between the
hot end and the cool end? _____ **4–5°C**

HUMIDITY

What is the humidity? _____ **45%**

Is there a humidity gauge? _____ **Yes**

How is it provided? _____ **Damp moss and the lizard is lightly**
sprayed each day while it is young

DÉCOR

What substrate is used? _____ **Calci-sand**

How deep is the substrate? _____ **2 cm**

How frequently is the vivarium cleaned out? ___ **When it is dirty**

What cleaning solution is used? _____ **Wipe out 1**
terrarium cleaner

Describe the hide box/es _____ **Ceramic hide 'rock'**

Is there a covered, damp moss/peat container? _____ **Yes**

What other items of décor are there? (Rocks, branches,

drain pipes, plants – plastic or real etc) _____ **Proprietary wood**

sculptures, mopani wood, branches, rocks

FEEDING

List **all** food items given including quantity and frequency *or*

complete the diet sheet (If fruit & vegetables

list each type) _____ **A selection of fruit & vegetables**

& 2 crickets daily

How often is the animal fed? _____ **Twice daily**

What supplements are provided and

how often? _____ **Vionate every day**

If feeding with insects, how do you ensure the

supplement is delivered? _____ **Crickets are fed by hand**

What are the insects fed on? _____ **Pro-grub cricket diet**

What size is the water container? _____ **Small bowl about**

3″ diameter

SOCIAL GROUPING

What other individuals of the same or different

species share the accommodation? _____ **More baby Bearded**

Dragons

How many are there of each

and of what sex _____ **Four in total. Sex unknown**

Do they tend to mix with or ignore each other? _____ **Both**

Is there at least one hide per individual? _____ **Yes**

COOLING DOWN

Please describe fully the process of cooling down,

length of cooling & warming back up. _____ **Too young**

for cooling down yet

ANY OTHER COMMENTS

_____

_____

_____

_____

_____

_____

_____

_____

COMMENTS

ANIMAL'S DETAILS

- This is a very young animal; usually a breeder will not let a hatchling go until it is a little older and they are sure it is doing well.
- The fact that it has not been wormed yet is not necessarily a problem. Normally I would not have wormed an animal this young unless there was a related problem.

HOUSING

VIVARIUM

- Whilst this is a good size for an adult, a hatchling requires much smaller accommodation. When young, most reptiles are very conscious of the fact that they could become dinner for just about anything. At this age a smaller vivarium will allow them to feel much more secure.
- I would want more detail about the size and position of the ventilation grills. Admittedly, this is irrelevant if they are going to change the accommodation, but when the animal is older this vivarium will once again be operational.

LIGHTING

- If Poggy cannot come into contact with the spotlight/basking light then a guard is not essential, however, I would advise one anyway to be on the safe side.
- Obviously it is too soon to have replaced the UV but the owner should be questioned to ascertain that they know how often it needs changing.

HEATING

- As previously stated, I do not usually recommend the use of heat mats inside the vivarium and would advise an alternative method of heating.
- For such a young individual, it is best to keep the temperature fluctuation minimal. Ideally, for this species it should not go below 26°C at night. The daytime and basking temperatures are fine. However, the smaller the vivarium the more difficult it is to get the necessary temperature range without the use of, for example a moss container or clay drainpipe to provide cooler areas.

DÉCOR

- 'Calci-sand' is supposed to be digestible but there have been reports that it has caused impaction in adult animals. In young animals this risk is increased as they do tend to take in a lot of substrate with their food, which is necessarily chopped up very finely. Perhaps a less interesting but safer substrate such as newspaper is advisable while it is this young.

FEEDING

- The list of food items prompts further questioning: exactly what fruit and vegetables are offered? I am looking for a good variety.
- What size are the crickets? Bearded dragons seem particularly susceptible to impaction due to eating crickets that are too large. This can result in partial paralysis (hind leg extension).

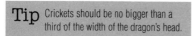

Tip Crickets should be no bigger than a third of the width of the dragon's head.

- Feeding twice daily at this age is correct. As the animal gets older this can be reduced to once daily.

- The manufacturer states that 'Vionate' is suitable for a range of animals but this does not make it appropriate for reptiles; they should be given a reptile-specific supplement.

SOCIAL GROUPING

Further questioning is necessary to establish that the owner is aware of the following:

1   Close observation is essential when housing young or hatchlings together in order to monitor each individual's progress.
2   If young bearded dragons are kept together there is a risk of bullying or intimidation by larger individuals. To reduce this, only youngsters of a similar size should be housed together. Smaller ones are better off on their own if there are no others of the same size and they are being bullied.

COOLING DOWN

- The owner is quite right, they are too young for cooling down and, depending on how the animal is progressing, may not be ready until their 2nd year. It should be ascertained that the owner is aware of the correct procedure for cooling down.

HISTORY

TORTOISES

[IF THE TORTOISE IS KEPT IN A VIVARIUM INSIDE THE HOUSE USE THE HISTORY FORM FOR SNAKES & LIZARDS]

ANIMAL'S DETAILS

Name _____ **Archimedes**

Species _____ **Spur-thighed tortoise**

Sex _____ **Male**

Where did you get it from? _____ **Rescued**

Approximate age _____ **30 yrs**

How long have you had it? _____ **2 yrs**

When and with what was it

last wormed? _____ **1 yr ago (last summer)**

HOUSING

HOUSE

During inclement weather is the tortoise shut in its house or does it still have access to the outside? _____ **Has access**
Describe the housing and run. Include approximate size, construction materials and a diagram if applicable. (If there is more than one accommodation type provided, fill in a separate form for each.) _____ **Fibreglass rabbit hutch measuring 3′ × 2′ (1 m × 61 cm). The inside sleeping side has a hay bed. The hutch is inside an enclosed run measuring 6′ × 12′ (1.8 × 3.6 m), which is part shrubs and part grass.**

LIGHTING

Is there any UV provision? (State type used and
how frequently it is changed) _____ **No**
How high above 'tortoise level' is it placed? _____ **N/A**
Is there a spotlight/basking light? (State type & wattage) ____ **No**
For how long are the lights on each day? _____ **N/A**

HEATING

What type of heater is used? _____ **None**
Does it have a guard around it? _____ **N/A**
Is it connected to a thermostat? _____ **N/A**
What is the background temperature?

Day	Night
Whatever the temperature is outside	

What is the temperature variation between
the hot and cold sections? _____ **N/A**
What is the temperature under the spotlight/
basking light? _____ **N/A**
What type of thermometer is used? _____ **None**

DECOR

What substrate is used? _____ **Newspaper & hay**
How frequently is it cleaned out? _____ **Fortnightly**
What cleaning solution is used? _____ **None**
Describe the hide box/es _____ **None**
If there a special area for egg laying, describe it? _____ **N/A**

FEEDING

List **all** types of food items fed and state approximately how
often each is given. _____ **Red apple, broccoli & leaves,
cucumber – daily, lettuce, cabbage,
greens, dandelion leaves, pear, peas,**

spinach – one of these every other day,
peaches, plum, banana – one a week
Milupa – stomach tubed at the beginning
of summer every third day

State approximately how much is given on a
daily basis _____ **As much as he will eat, which is not much.**
What supplements are given and how often? ____ **Nutrobal – daily**

SOCIAL GROUPING

What other individuals of the same or different
species share the accommodation? (State how
many there are of each and of what sex) _____ **None**
Describe how they interact with each other _____ **N/A**

HIBERNATION

If you provide a gradual cooling down
prior to hibernation, please describe the
process _____ **Natural weather & light conditions**
For how long is food withheld prior to
entering hibernation? _____ **2 weeks**
Do you worm the tortoise prior to hibernation? _____ **No**
How do you ensure adequate bodyweight prior to
hibernation? _____ **Weigh**
Describe the hibernation accommodation and
siting in detail _____ **Inner box with shredded newspaper**
surrounded by polystyrene balls contained
in an outer box. Raised above the garage floor.
How often do you check the tortoise
during hibernation? _____ **Monthly**
At the end of hibernation do you wake the tortoise
yourself or allow it to wake up on its own? _____ **On its own**

If it wakes up by itself, how do you know

when it has done so? _____ **Check every few days**

at the beginning of spring

Please describe what you do immediately

the tortoise has woken up and for the

following few days _____ **Bath in warm water to encourage**

to drink. When active, force feed watery

food e.g. cucumber

ANY OTHER COMMENTS

Also allowed in the rest of the garden under supervision for about 30 min. on most days.

Sometimes brought into the house, he will sit on a hot water bottle for a while then wander around.

COMMENTS

I always find commenting on tortoise husbandry a little tricky. On the one hand, there may be glaring errors, on the other, the tortoise may have been kept successfully like this for many years.

If I have experienced, or heard about a problem with a particular procedure, I may decide not to run the risk of using it. For example, many tortoises will wake up during their hibernation, then go back to sleep again and reawaken with no trouble at all. But there have been instances when the tortoise has not had sufficient energy to wake up properly for the 2nd time and this has caused problems or even death.

My policy, therefore, is to make tentative suggestions, **unless** there is a problem, then I will point out any errors.

In this instance, the problem was that the tortoise was not eating well and never had done during the two years he had been with his new owners.

ANIMAL'S DETAILS

- The type of wormer has not been stated so I would need to know this.
- It is wormed annually (which is more than most), however, twice yearly would be better.

HOUSING
HOUSE

- The size of the house and run are fine but fibreglass offers no thermal retention at all. This might not be a problem if there was some wood or other material surrounding it, but there is no mention of this.

LIGHTING

- If there is regular access to the outside the need for UV provision is arguable, but it should be ascertained how often the tortoise actually goes outside. The British summer, unfortunately, can be rather erratic. If the tortoise chooses not to venture out on rainy, damp or overcast days there may not be much exposure to the sun.
- Again, because of the vagaries of the weather a basking spot is pretty much essential, either inside the house or somewhere in the run or both.

HEATING

- With no subsidiary heating at all it is not surprising that the tortoise does not eat well. He probably rarely reaches his P.B.T. and is therefore not inclined to eat, and what is eaten will take much longer to metabolise than it should.

DÉCOR

- The fact that there is not a hide box is probably not significant. Provided that there is sufficient hay inside the hutch for the tortoise to 'burrow' into he will feel just as secure. He also has access to the garden shrubs where he could probably hide if he wanted to, although he might get rather cold.
- If the hutch does not get dirty it is probably not necessary to use a cleaning solution every time the substrate is changed, but it is still a good idea to clean it periodically.

FEEDING

- The variety is not too bad. Probably, he is somewhat fussy as to what he will eat at the moment; once he has started eating properly the variety should, hopefully, increase. I would suggest that tortoise pellets also be included in the diet.

- Broccoli should not be fed on a daily basis as it is high in oxalates and can interfere with calcium metabolism.
- Tube feeding with 'Milupa' is a very common mistake. It should be remembered that this is a food designed for mammals and includes milk powder. Tortoises do not have the ability to digest milk. A couple of alternatives would be:

1   Tins/jars of pure fruit or vegetable baby food. Those that do not contain added preservatives, artificial flavours, colours, salt, sugar, gluten, milk, egg, etc. can be watered down to a suitable consistency for stomach tubing. They are readily available from most places that sell baby food.
2   If you are really keen you can purée your own concoction of fruit/vegetables.

HIBERNATION

- Withholding food for only two weeks prior to hibernation, especially if there is not additional heating, is not long enough to ensure that the digestive tract is completely empty. At least a month is required under normal circumstances.
- Worming has already been mentioned.
- The hibernation accommodation is one of the areas that may take some persuasion as the owners have used the current method for the last two years and the tortoise has not died.
- Shredded newspaper is fine but tends to compact down quickly; paper that has been through a shredding machine tends to hold its shape better.
- The polystyrene balls for insulation between the two boxes is good.

- I would want to know what the outer box is made of. Is it rodent proof?
- Is the tortoise's weight monitored?
- Questions resulting from keeping it in the garage:
  - How is the temperature monitored?
  - What happens if the temperature goes below 0°C or starts to creep up towards 10°C?
  - What are the levels of carbon monoxide? (In other words, when the car is started first thing in the morning, is the engine left running to warm up?)
- Bathing the tortoise when it has woken up is good but I do not personally hold with force-feeding. I believe that the stress caused and the amount of energy the tortoise uses up fighting the process are more detrimental than leaving it alone. If it is not eating within a few days of emerging from hibernation, stomach tubing is a better option.

4 PHOTOGRAPHS OF INJURIES CAUSED THROUGH INAPPROPRIATE HUSBANDRY

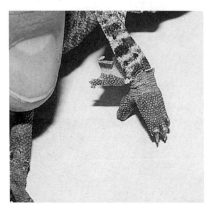

Fig. 4.1 It is not uncommon for lizards to have difficulty sloughing their feet, often but not necessarily due to the humidity being low Reproduced, with permission, from *Reptile Medicine and Surgery* by Mader. Saunders (1996)

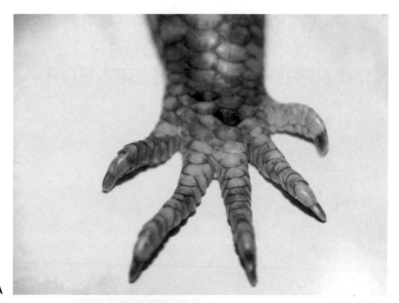

A

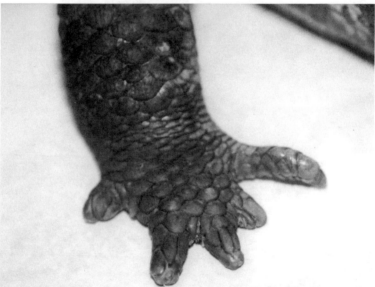

B

Fig. 4.2 Photograph **A** shows a normal foot, photograph **B** shows the effect of insufficient humidity which caused difficulty in sloughing the skin off the toes properly and resulted in parts of them being lost.

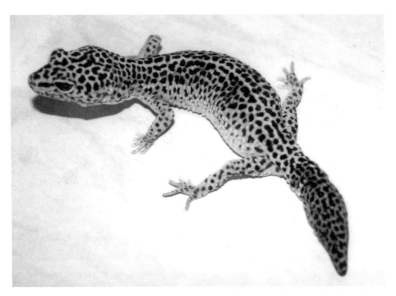

Fig. 4.3 Many lizards have the ability to shed their tails as a defence mechanism. In captivity this is most often caused through incorrect handling or fighting. Hatchlings being afraid of just about anything, may sometimes be a little over-enthusiastic about dropping their tails. This photograph shows a tail after it has regrown

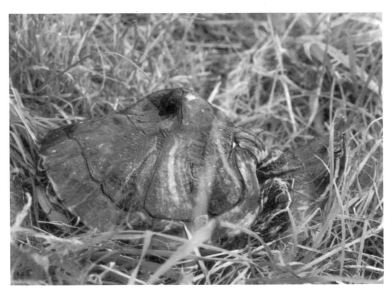

Fig. 4.4 The misshapen shell of a red-eared terrapin, probably caused by insufficient UV provision or lack of correct vitamin/mineral supplementation

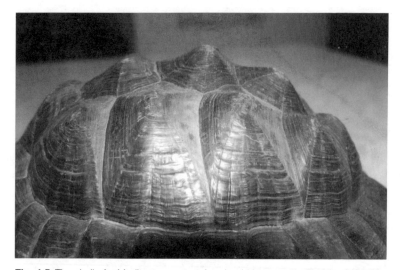

Fig. 4.5 The shell of a Mediterranean tortoise should be smooth. The doming of the individual scutes shown here is usually caused by too rapid growth as a hatchling or when young.

The diet of a captive tortoise is far better than that of a wild one which, for the most part, is for the good. However, for hatchlings and youngsters less protein and a good vitamin/mineral supplement is essential, otherwise the shell will grow too rapidly resulting in this doming effect and/or the condition known as 'soft shell', which is caused by a lack of calcium.

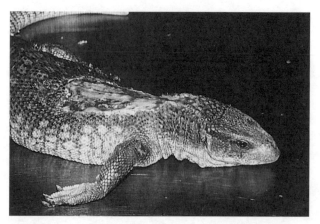

Fig. 4.6 Burns caused by an unguarded heat lamp. Reproduced, with permission, from *Reptile Medicine and Surgery* by Mader. Saunders (1996)

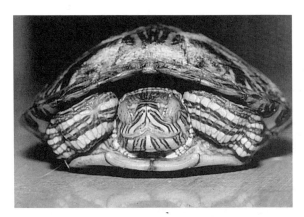

Fig. 4.7 Advanced hypovitaminosis A. Conjunctival and orbital gland swelling causes the globe to be completely covered with dysplastic tissue. Reproduced, with permission, from *Reptile Medicine and Surgery* by Mader. Saunders (1996)

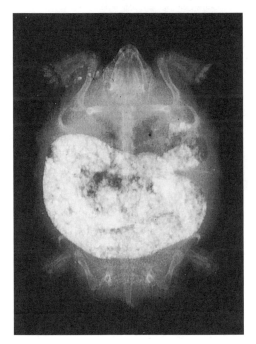

Fig. 4.8 Intestinal impaction due to ingesting the sand substrate this tortoise was kept on. Reproduced, with permission, from *Reptile Medicine and Surgery* by Mader. Saunders (1996)

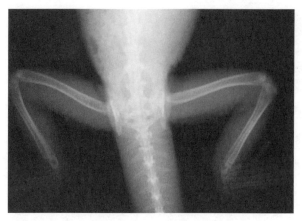

Fig. 4.9 Common iguana with normal bone density. Reproduced, with permission, from *Reptile Medicine and Surgery* by Mader. Saunders (1996)

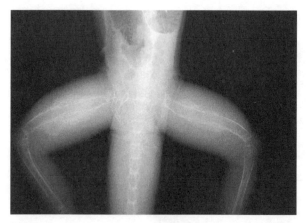

Fig. 4.10 Common iguana with metabolic bone disease. Reproduced, with permission, from *Reptile Medicine and Surgery* by Mader. Saunders (1996)

APPENDIX 1

WEEKLY DIET SHEET

SPECIES ———————

DAY	FOOD/S	AMOUNT	SUPPLEMENT (STATE TYPE)
Monday			
Tuesday			
Wednesday			
Thursday			
Friday			
Saturday			
Sunday			

APPENDIX 2

FLOW CHART FOR IDENTIFYING CAUSES OF FEEDING PROBLEMS IN SNAKES

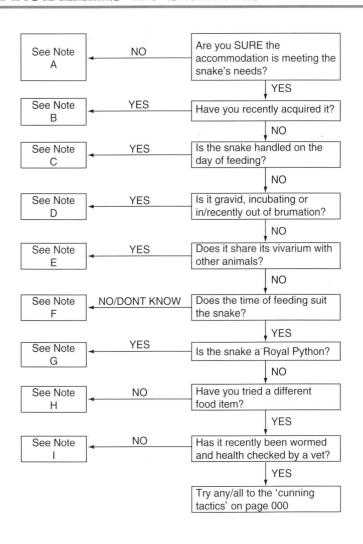

See Note A	◄ NO	Are you SURE the accommodation is meeting the snake's needs?
		↓ YES
See Note B	◄ YES	Have you recently acquired it?
		↓ NO
See Note C	◄ YES	Is the snake handled on the day of feeding?
		↓ NO
See Note D	◄ YES	Is it gravid, incubating or in/recently out of brumation?
		↓ NO
See Note E	◄ YES	Does it share its vivarium with other animals?
		↓ NO
See Note F	◄ NO/DONT KNOW	Does the time of feeding suit the snake?
		↓ YES
See Note G	◄ YES	Is the snake a Royal Python?
		↓ NO
See Note H	◄ NO	Have you tried a different food item?
		↓ YES
See Note I	◄ NO	Has it recently been wormed and health checked by a vet?
		↓ YES
		Try any/all to the 'cunning tactics' on page 000

NOTES:

A Obviously, if the set up is not right and the snake does not feel happy and secure it will not feed. Establish that lighting, temperatures, etc. are correct and there is somewhere for it to hide.

B When a snake is newly acquired it will need to have a 'settling in' period. During this time it should be handled as little as possible and not offered food immediately, until it is used to its new regime.

C Handling can be quite stressful for some individuals and a stressed snake will probably refuse to eat. If you have a snake that does not mind being handled this probably will not be an issue, however, it is worth eliminating the possibility.

D At certain times in an individual snake's yearly cycle it may not eat as part of its natural behaviour pattern. Some females will not eat for a part or even all of the length of the time they are gravid and in those species that incubate, such as pythons, she may well refuse to eat during this time. Obviously, if a snake is in a cooling down period it should not be fed, but even if you have not cooled it down, if it would naturally do so in the wild it may refuse food for the natural duration. Also, when many species come out of brumation they only have one thing on their mind – mating – and eating tends to be ignored for a time.

E As a rule, snakes should not be fed in the presence of other snakes. There may be a tussle over a food item and if two snakes latch onto opposite ends of a mouse one may end up trying to eat the other! Another possibility, although less likely, is that the presence of another snake may inhibit the other's feeding response.

Therefore, split individuals into separate vivariums before feeding. However, in some instances individuals who are happy with their companions and in their surroundings may object to being moved or separated and this in itself may cause them to refuse. In this instance the UTMOST CARE must be taken when feeding and the snakes must remain under observation all the time there is a food item in the vivarium.

F Find out when the snake is active in the wild, that is, whether it is nocturnal, diurnal or crepuscular (this may change at different times of the year) and feed it at a time that suits its natural habits, not yours. Also bear in mind any external stimulus that may occur at feeding time. For example, if it is in a busy room where there is a lot of activity it may be put off feeding.

G Royal pythons, particularly wild caught individuals, are notorious for being difficult feeders. As well as trying all the other suggestions, you could try offering gerbils for which they have a particular penchant.

H The food item may be too big or too small so try a different size, perhaps a small rabbit instead of large rat, for instance. Alternatively, the snake may have become choosy or fed up with the same thing, so try a different type, e.g. rat pup instead of small mouse. A word of **warning** though: it is best to avoid chicks and chickens as these may become 'addictive' and the snake may end up refusing everything else. Whilst this may not be a problem with some types of food, the nutritional value of chicken is not as good as other foods and if fed solely on these the snake may develop a nutritional deficiency.

I Routine worming should be carried out twice a year. If the snake has not been wormed regularly it may develop a heavy parasite burden, which could become a serious problem. Anorexia may be one of the symptoms.

If a snake has stopped eating it would be as well to get it checked over by a vet. Obviously, if there is a health problem the sooner it is treated the better the chance of recovery, and if it transpires that it is healthy then at least you have eliminated the possibility of illness.

CUNNING TACTICS FOR
FEEDING PROBLEM SNAKES

If the snake is being fed on mice, try a different colour.

• Some snakes are colour prejudiced. For example, one might simply refuse to eat white mice but will happily take black ones.

Leave snake overnight in a small container, with food.

• It is possible that the snake does not feel secure enough. In this case placing it in a small container with a suitable hide, and so on, may give it the sense of security it needs in order to feed. Should this method prove to be successful, you will need to reassess the vivarium set-up to ensure that it does feel secure in its home.

Blood or pith the food item.

• Chop the top of the head off the prey item exposing the brain, or cut it elsewhere allowing blood to seep out. This enhances the smell of the item and makes it more appealing.

Use the 'wiggle & drag' technique.

• This is where an attempt is made to fool the snake into thinking the prey is still alive. (Snakes are not very bright.) To do this, the food is wiggled around and dragged back and forth in front of the snake. The movement may trigger the strike response.

Warm the prey up to body temperature.

• This is particularly important for species that possess 'heat pits', such as pythons. In the wild snakes generally only eat live prey which would naturally be warm. Heating the food to body temperature therefore simulates a more realistic approach. NB, do not attempt to heat the prey in a microwave oven as there is a tendency for them to explode.

Avoid direct handling of the food.

• Use tongs or rubber gloves whenever handling the prey (including when defrosting) to avoid getting human scent on the food, which may be off-putting for the snake.

The following methods should only be attempted if all the above have been tried unsuccessfully. Please read the accompanying notes carefully.

Freshly killed prey

• Offering prey that has recently been killed rather than previously frozen may be more tempting, especially if it is still warm and/or bloodied. If this method meets with success it is advisable to attempt to get the snake onto defrosted food as soon as possible as this is not a particularly convenient way of feeding.

Force-feeding

• This should only be attempted when veterinary opinion is such that drastic measures are necessary i.e. the snake is in danger of becoming undernourished. There are two basic methods of force-feeding:

1   The first one is to literally try to force the food into the snake's mouth and get it to swallow. However, the potential to harm the snake during this process, coupled with the fact that the amount of stress caused outweighs any possible benefit, means that this method is **not recommended**.
2   The alternative, and **preferred**, method is to stomach-tube the snake using either liquidised prey or an appropriate baby food (one that is meat-flavoured and without milk, salt, sugar, etc).

NB Force-feeding should only be attempted under veterinary direction and by someone experienced in this method.

Live-feeding

- A vexed subject! Contrary to popular belief, live feeding is not illegal in this country. The law that applies in this instance states that it is illegal to cause 'unnecessary suffering'. Allowing a snake to starve to death could be considered as unnecessary suffering and live feeding is, after all, only mimicking what would occur in the wild.

There are a few do's and don'ts to be followed if attempting this method:

1   Do not leave the prey in with the snake for too long; if a snake is going to strike it will be sooner rather than later. The exact length of time will depend on the individual but, as a guide, about 15–30 minutes should be enough to determine if the snake is interested. Leaving it for longer could be deemed as unnecessary suffering to the prey which may also start to nibble on the snake.
2   Evidence must be available to show that this is a LAST RESORT and that every effort was made to entice the snake to eat before trying live-feeding.
3   Continued attempts must be made to get the snake to eat dead food.

Many people feel that this method is a step too far and will not participate in live-feeding. It is a matter on which each individual must decide for him/herself.

Table 1 Biological data – snakes, lizards, tortoises and terrapins

SPECIES	PBT[a]	AVERAGE CLUTCH SIZE	INCUBATION[b]	SEXUAL MATURITY[c]	AVERAGE LIFE SPAN
Red Eared Terrapin	25–32°C	4–6	8–12 weeks at 26–30°C	3–4 years	30–40 years
Spur Thighed Tortoise	30–35°C	4–8 (1–2 per year)	2–3 months at 26–30°C	6–15 years	50–100 years
Corn snake	25–32°C	5–30 (1–2 per year)	55–72 days at 25–30°C	1½–2 years	15–20 years
Royal Python	27–32°C	4–10	2–3 months at 28–30°C	1–2 years	20–30 years
Leopard Gecko	26–30°C	2 (5–6 per year)	55–65 days at 26–30°C	1½–2 years	15–20 years
Green Iguana	30–35°C	12–40	3–4 months at 28–30°C	1½–2 years	15–20 years
Bearded Dragon	27–38°C	15–25 (2–3) per year	2–3 months at 28–30°C	1–2 years	10–20 years[d]

[a]PBT   –Preferred body temperature. Includes basking temperature

[b]Incubation   –The higher the temperature (within the range) the quicker the incubation

–Lizards & chelonia are subject to temperature-dependant sex determination. Lizard eggs incubated at the higher end of the range will be predominantly male and those at the lower end predominantly female. For chelonia, this is reversed

[c]Sexual maturity   –This usually relates to size rather than age.

[d]Bearded dragons tend to have a shortened life span as they are commonly overfed, particularly if the proportion of insects (or meat) in the diet is too high

Table 2 Biological data – amphibians

SPECIES	PBT[a]	AVERAGE CLUTCH SIZE	GESTATION/ INCUBATION[b]	METAMORPHOSIS (approx. start – finish)	SEXUAL MATURITY[c]	AVERAGE LIFE SPAN
Fire-bellied Toad	26–28°C	40–100 (1–2 per year)	3–5 days at 21–24°C	3–5 weeks at 24°C	1–2 years	12–15 years
Ornate Horned Frog	26–28°C	1000–2000 (1–2 per year)	1–3 days at 24–28°C	2–4 weeks at 24°C	1½–2 years	7–10 years
White's Tree Frog	25–30°C	500–1000 (3–4 per year)	1–2 days at 26–30°C	3–8 weeks at 26–30°C	1–2 years	10–15 years
European Fire Salamander	17–20°C	20–70 **LIVE LARVAE** (1–2 per year)	2–5 months at 15–20°C	2–4 months at 15–20°C	2–4 years	12–20 years

[a]PBT   –Preferred body temperature. Includes basking temperature (where relevant)

[b]Incubation   –The higher the temperature (within the range) the quicker the incubation

[c]Sexual Maturity   –This is usually related to size rather than age

INDEX

Index

Index

Index

Multimedia CD-ROM
Single User License Agreement

1. NOTICE. WE ARE WILLING TO LICENSE THE MULTI-MEDIA PROGRAM PRODUCT TITLED "*The Really Useful Handbook of Reptile Husbandry*" ("MULTIMEDIA PROGRAM") TO YOU ONLY ON THE CONDITION THAT YOU ACCEPT ALL OF THE TERMS CONTAINED IN THIS LICENSE AGREEMENT. PLEASE READ THIS LICENSE AGREEMENT CAREFULLY BEFORE OPENING THE SEALED DISK PACKAGE. BY OPENING THAT PACKAGE YOU AGREE TO BE BOUND BY THE TERMS OF THIS AGREEMENT. IF YOU DO NOT AGREE TO THESE TERMS WE ARE UNWILLING TO LICENSE THE MULTIMEDIA PROGRAME TO YOU, AND YOU SHOULD NOT OPEN THE DISK PACKAGE. IN SUCH CASE, PROMPTLY RETURN THE UNOPENED DISK PACKAGE AND ALL OTHER MATERIAL IN THIS PACKAGE, ALONG WITH PROOF OF PAYMENT, TO THE AUTHORISED DEALER FROM WHOM YOU OBTAINED IT FOR A FULL REFUND OF THE PRICE YOU PAID.

2. **Ownership and License**. This is a license agreement and NOT an agreement for sale. It permits you to use one copy of the MULTIMEDIA PROGRAM on a single computer. The MULTIMEDIA PROGRAM and its contents are owned by us or our licensors, and are protected by U.S. and international copyright laws. Your rights to use the MULTIMEDIA PROGRAM are specified in this Agreement, and we retain all rights not expressly granted to you in this Agreement.
   - You may use one copy of the MULTIMEDIA PROGRAM on a single computer
   - After you have installed the MULTIMEDIA PROGRAM on your computer, you may use the MULTIMEDIA PROGRAM on a different computer only if you first delete the files installed by the installation program from the first computer.
   - You may not copy any portion of the MULTIMEDIA PROGRAM to your computer hard disk or any other media other than printing out or downloading non-substantial portions of the text and images in the MULTIMEDIA PROGRAM for your own internal informational use.
   - Your may not copy any of the documentation or other printed materials accompanying the MULTIMEDIA PROGRAM.

Neither concurrent use on two or more computers nor use in a local area network or other network is permitted without separate authorisation and the payment of additional license fees.

3. **Transfer and Other Restrictions**. You may not rent, lend, or lease this MULTIMEDIA PROGRAM. Save as permitted by law, you may not and you may not permit others to (a) disassemble, decompile, or otherwise derive source code from the software included in the MULTIMEDIA PROGRAM (the "Software"), (b) reverse engineer the Software, (c) modify or prepare derivative works of the MULTIMEDIA PROGRAM (d) use the Software in an on-line system, or (e) use the MULTIMEDIA PROGRAM in any manner that infringes on the intellectual property or other rights of another party.

   However, you may transfer this license to use the MULTIMEDIA PROGRAM to another party on a permanent basis by transferring this copy of the License Agreement, the MULTIMEDIA PROGRAM, and all documentation. Such transfer of possession terminates your license from us. Such other party shall be licensed under the terms of this Agreement upon its acceptance of this Agreement by its initial use of the MULTIMEDIA PROGRAM. If you transfer the MULTIMEDIA PROGRAM, you must remove the installation files from your hard disk and you may not retain any copies of those files for your own use.

4. **Limited Warranty and Limitation of Liability**. For a period of sixty (60) days from the date you acquired the MULTIMEDIA PROGRAM from us or our authorised dealer, we warrant that the media containing the MULTIMEDIA PROGRAM will be free from defects that prevent you from installing the MULTIMEDIA PROGRAM on your computer. If the disk fails to conform to this warranty you may as your sole and exclusive remedy, obtain a replacement free of charge if you return the defective disk to us with a dated proof of purchase. Otherwise the MULTIMEDIA PROGRAM is licensed to you on an "AS IS" basis without any warranty of any nature.

   WE DO NOT WARRANT THAT THE MULTIMEDIA PROGRAM WILL MEET YOUR REQUIREMENTS OR THAT ITS OPERATION WILL BE UNINTERRUPTED OR ERROR-FREE. THE EXPRESS TERMS OF THIS AGREEMENT ARE IN LIEU OF

ALL WARRANTIES, CONDITIONS, UNDERTAKINGS, TERMS AND OBLIGATIONS IMPLIED BY STATUTE, COMMON LAW, TRADE USAGE, COURSE OF DEALING OR OTHERWISE ALL OF WHICH ARE HEREBY EXCLUDED TO THE FULLEST EXTENT PERMITTED BY LAW, INCLUDING THE IMPLIED WARRANTIES OF SATISFACTORY QUALITY AND FITNESS FOR A PARTICULAR PURPOSE.

WE SHALL NOT BE LIABLE FOR ANY DAMAGE OR LOSS OF ANY KIND (EXCEPT PERSONAL INJURY OR DEATH RESULTING FROM OUR NEGLIGENCE) ARISING OUT OF OR RESULTING FROM YOUR POSSESSION OR USE OF THE MULTIMEDIA PROGRAM (INCLUDING DATA LOSS OR CORRUPTION), REGARDLESS OF WHETHER SUCH LIABILITY IS BASED IN TORT, CONTRACT OR OTHERWISE AND INCLUDING, BUT NOT LIMITED TO, ACTUAL, SPECIAL, INDIRECT, INCIDENTAL OR CONSEQUENTIAL DAMAGES. IF THE FOREGOING LIMITATION IS HELD TO BE UNENFORCEABLE OUR MAXIMUM LIABILITY TO YOU SHALL NOT EXCEED THE AMOUNT OF THE LICENSE FEE PAID BY YOU FOR THE MULTIMEDIA PROGRAM. THE REMEDIES AVAILABLE TO YOU AGAINST US AND THE LICENSORS OF MATERIALS INCLUDED IN THE MULTIMEDIA PROGRAM ARE EXCLUSIVE.

5. **Termination.** This license and your right to use this MULTIMEDIA PROGRAM automatically terminate if you fail to comply with any provisions of this Agreement, destroy the copy of the MULTIMEDIA PROGRAM in your possession, or voluntarily return the MULTIMEDIA PROGRAM to us. Upon termination you will destroy all copies of the MULTIMEDIA PROGRAM and documentation.

6. **Miscellaneous Provisions.** This Agreement will be governed by and construed in accordance with English law and you hereby submit to the non-exclusive jurisdiction of the English Courts. This is the entire agreement between us relating to the MULTIMEDIA PROGRAM, and supersedes any prior purchase order, communications, advertising or representations concerning the contents of this package, No change or modification of this Agreement will be valid unless it is in writing and is signed by us.